AF478579

Prescription Drugs Under Medicare: The Legacy of the Task Force on Prescription Drugs

Prescription Drugs Under Medicare: The Legacy of the Task Force on Prescription Drugs has been co-published simultaneously as *Journal of Research in Pharmaceutical Economics,* Volume 10, Numbers 2/3 and 4 2001.

The *Journal of Research in Pharmaceutical Economics* Monographic "Separates"

Below is a list of "separates," which in serials librarianship means a special issue simultaneously published as a special journal issue or double-issue *and* as a "separate" hardbound monograph. (This is a format which we also call a "DocuSerial.")

"Separates" are published because specialized libraries or professionals may wish to purchase a specific thematic issue by itself in a format which can be separately cataloged and shelved, as opposed to purchasing the journal on an on-going basis. Faculty members may also more easily consider a "separate" for classroom adoption.

"Separates" are carefully classified separately with the major book jobbers so that the journal tie-in can be noted on new book order slips to avoid duplicate purchasing.

You may wish to visit Haworth's website at . . .

http://www.HaworthPress.com

. . . to search our online catalog for complete tables of contents of these separates and related publications.

You may also call 1-800-HAWORTH (outside US/Canada: 607-722-5857), or Fax 1-800-895-0582 (outside US/Canada: 607-771-0012), or e-mail at:

getinfo@haworthpressinc.com

Prescription Drugs Under Medicare: The Legacy of the Task Force on Prescription Drugs, edited by Mickey C. Smith, PhD (Vol. 10, No. 2/3 and No. 4, 2001). *The story of the very first serious Federal effort to study the feasibility of funding a drug benefits program for the elderly.*

Health Outcomes and Pharmaceutical Care: Measurement, Applications, and Initiatives, edited by Alan Escovitz, PhD, and Dev S. Pathak, DBA (Vol. 7, No. 4, 1996 and Vol. 8, No. 1, 1997). *"One of the few existing texts addressing both pharmaceutical care and health outcomes. . . . Excellent in its review of major issues in health outcomes and its breadth of coverage. Highly recommended for both academic libraries and personal libraries of those associated with managing or evaluating pharmacy programs."* (American Journal of Pharmaceutical Education)

Managed Competition and Pharmaceutical Care: A Challenge for the Profession, edited by Dev S. Pathak, DBA, and Alan Escovitz, PhD (Vol. 7, No. 1/2, 1996). *"A useful resource for anyone seeking to develop a better understanding of how regulatory and public policy strategies come about and how they are likely to affect the status quo of health care delivery and financing in the U.S."* (Pharmaceutical Research)

Prescription Drugs Under Medicare: The Legacy of the Task Force on Prescription Drugs

Mickey C. Smith
Editor

Prescription Drugs Under Medicare: The Legacy of the Task Force on Prescription Drugs has been co-published simultaneously as *Journal of Research in Pharmaceutical Economics,* Volume 10, Numbers 2/3 and 4 2001.

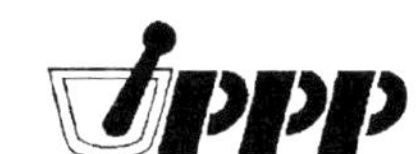

Pharmaceutical Products Press
An Imprint of
The Haworth Press, Inc.
New York • London • Oxford

Published by

Pharmaceutical Products Press®, 10 Alice Street, Binghamton, NY 13904-1580 USA

Pharmaceutical Products Press® is an imprint of The Haworth Press, Inc., 10 Alice Street, Binghamton, NY 13904-1580 USA.

Prescription Drugs Under Medicare: The Legacy of the Task Force on Prescription Drugs has been co-published simultaneously as *Journal of Research in Pharmaceutical Economics*™, Volume 10, Numbers 2/3 and 4 2001.

The development, preparation, and publication of this work has been undertaken with great care. However, the publisher, employees, editors, and agents of The Haworth Press and all imprints of The Haworth Press, Inc., including The Haworth Medical Press® and Pharmaceutical Products Press®, are not responsible for any errors contained herein or for consequences that may ensue from use of materials or information contained in this work. Opinions expressed by the author(s) are not necessarily those of The Haworth Press, Inc.

Cover design by Thomas J. Mayshock Jr.

Library of Congress Cataloging-in-Publication Data

Prescription drugs under medicare : the legacy of the Task Force on Prescription Drugs / Mickey C. Smith, editor.
      p. cm.
  "Prescription drugs under medicare: the legacy of the Task Force on Prescription Drugs has been co-published simultaneously as Journal of research in pharmaceutical economics, Volume 10, Numbers 2/3 and 4 2001."
  Includes bibliographical references and index.
  ISBN 0-7890-1306-1 (hard : alk. paper) – ISBN 0-7890-1307-X (pbk. : alk. paper)
  1. Medicare. 2. Prescription pricing–United States. 3. Insurance, Pharmaceutical services–United States. I. Smith, Mickey C. II. United States. Task Force on Prescription Drugs. III. Journal of research in pharmaceutical economics.

RA412.3 .P73 2001
362.1′782′0973–dc21
                                         00-068834

Indexing, Abstracting & Website/Internet Coverage

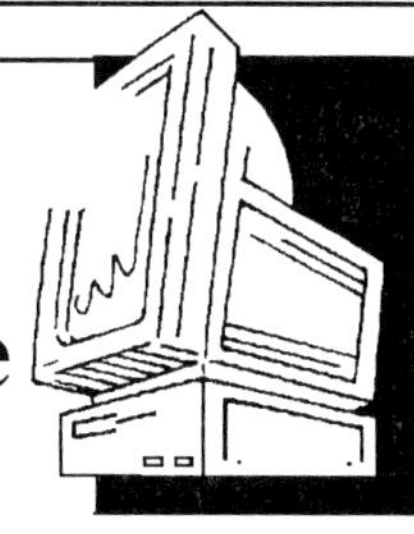

This section provides you with a list of major indexing & abstracting services. That is to say, each service began covering this periodical during the year noted in the right column. Most Websites which are listed below have indicated that they will either post, disseminate, compile, archive, cite or alert their own Website users with research-based content from this work. (This list is as current as the copyright date of this publication.)

Abstracting, Website/Indexing Coverage .... Year When Coverage Began

- *Adis International Ltd* 1992

- *Biosciences Information Service of Biological Abstracts (BIOSIS)* 1991

- *BUBL INFORMATION SERVICE: An Internet-based Information Service for the UK higher education community <URL: http://bubl.ac.uk/>* 1995

- *CNPIEC Reference Guide: Chinese National Directory of Foreign Periodicals* 1995

- *EconLit, on CD-ROM, and e-JEL* 1992

- *EMBASE/Excerpta Medica Secondary Publishing Division <URL: http://www.elsevier.nl>* 1996

- *FINDEX <www.publist.com>* 1999

- *Index to Periodical Articles Related to Law* 1991

- *International Pharmaceutical Abstracts* 1991

- *Medical Benefits* 1992

- *Pharmacy Business* 1991

(continued)

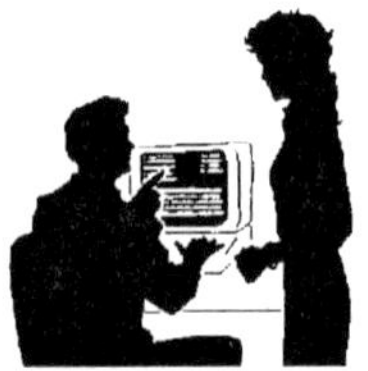

Prescription Drugs
Under Medicare:
The Legacy of the Task Force
on Prescription Drugs

CONTENTS

ABOUT THE EDITOR

Mickey C. Smith, Ph.D., is a highly acclaimed researcher/writer with an international reputation in the field of pharmaceutical marketing. He was named Mississippi's Professor of the Year for 1993, an honor conferred annually on one college instructor per state by the Council for Advancement and Support of Education (CASE) in Washington.

Dr. Smith joined the University of Mississippi in 1966 and began a long career of scholarship that has included ten books on pharmaceutical marketing and patient care. He is the principal author and editor of *Pharmaceutical Marketing: Strategy and Cases*, the only textbook of its kind. He has consulted with numerous pharmaceutical firms and government agencies and has published over 350 articles in over 100 different research and professional journals. As Executive Editor of Pharmaceutical Products Press, an imprint of The Haworth Press, Inc., Dr. Smith is also editor of the *Journal of Research in Pharmaceutical Economics* and the *Journal of Pharmaceutical Marketing & Management*.

He is currently Research Professor in Health Services Research at the University of Mississippi. His various awards include the Research Achievement Award from the Academy of Pharmaceutical Sciences, the Rho Chi national lecture award, the first-ever Lyman Award, the first-ever Distinguished Educator Award from the American Association of Colleges of Pharmacy, and, from the University of Mississippi, a Barnard Distinguished Professorship and the Burlington-Northern Teacher of the Year Award. Dr. Smith also holds a joint professorship with the University of Mississippi School of Business Administration.

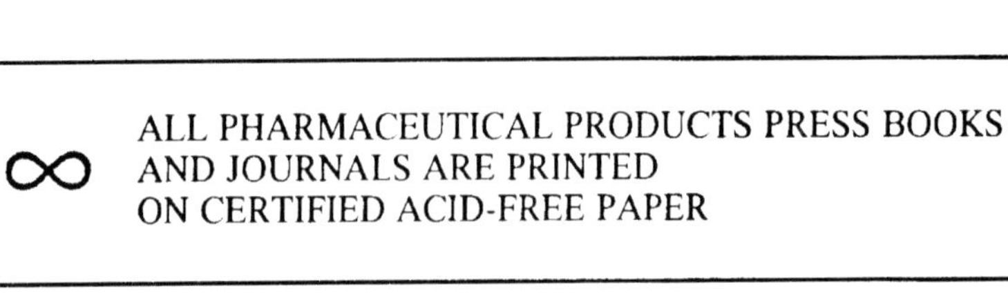

Introduction

The year 2000 may see (or have seen, by the time this is read) federal provision of outpatient prescription drugs as a benefit of the Medicare program.

Or it may not.

Regardless of the outcome of the deliberations on the subject during the first election of the new millennium, there is value, we believe, in reviewing events and efforts in previous attempts to provide drug benefits to the elderly population. That is the reason for this collection of materials.

The largest part of what follows is centered around the report of the Task Force on Prescription Drugs, the most extensive effort ever by the federal government to understand the nature of prescription medication use, especially among the elderly, in the United States. The Task Force Final Report is reprinted in its entirety, along with comments by two of its primary architects, Dr. T. Donald Rucker and Dr. Philip Lee.

The work of the Task Force was ultimately reviewed by a special committee (the "Dunlop Committee"). Excerpts from that review and selected comments by members of the committee are also reproduced here.

Readers will note that there was consensus, following such extensive study, that a Medicare prescription drug benefit plan was both needed and practical. But no such benefit plan was provided. It was not until 1988 that Congress passed legislation providing the long-awaited benefit program. The Medicare Catastrophic Protection Act of 1987 included prescription medications. In 1989, the Medicare Cata-

[Haworth co-indexing entry note]: "Introduction." Smith, Mickey C. Co-published simultaneously in *Journal of Research in Pharmaceutical Economics* (Pharmaceutical Products Press, an imprint of The Haworth Press, Inc.) Vol. 10, No. 2/3, 2001, pp. 1-2; and: *Prescription Drugs Under Medicare: The Legacy of the Task Force on Prescription Drugs* (ed: Mickey C. Smith) Pharmaceutical Products Press, an imprint of The Haworth Press, Inc., 2001, pp. 1-2. Single or multiple copies of this article are available for a fee from The Haworth Document Delivery Service [1-800-342-9678, 9:00 a.m. - 5:00 p.m. (EST). E-mail address: getinfo@haworthpressinc.com].

strophic Coverage *Repeal* Act was passed. The story of this extraordinary set of actions by Congress could fill a book. We will be able to provide only some of the flavor of the time.

The final component of this collection is a 1997 report, "A Framework for Research and Evaluation into the Effects of Managed Care on the Pharmaceutical Marketplace." In comment on the report, its authors hark back to the work for the Task Force and suggest how intervening events and possible developments in the future can be used.

We believe strongly that the information contained herein, some of which is not easily accessible, is essential to an understanding of how the stage was set for the debates of the year 2000. We hope readers will agree.

Mickey C. Smith

Editor's Note

Dr. T. Donald Rucker was one of the principal architects of the work and publication of the work of the Task Force on Prescription Drugs. After leaving the Social Security Administration, Dr. Rucker embarked on a career in pharmacy education. He has been honored for his research in pharmaceutical economics and known for his leadership in rational drug therapy. We asked him to author the first paper in the inaugural issue of the *Journal of Research in Pharmaceutical Economics*. It is reproduced here.

[Haworth co-indexing entry note]: "Editor's Note." Smith, Mickey C. Co-published simultaneously in *Journal of Research in Pharmaceutical Economics* (Pharmaceutical Products Press, an imprint of The Haworth Press, Inc.) Vol. 10, No. 2/3, 2001, p. 3; and: *Prescription Drugs Under Medicare: The Legacy of the Task Force on Prescription Drugs* (ed: Mickey C. Smith) Pharmaceutical Products Press, an imprint of The Haworth Press, Inc., 2001, p. 3. Single or multiple copies of this article are available for a fee from The Haworth Document Delivery Service [1-800-342-9678, 9:00 a.m. - 5:00 p.m. (EST). E-mail address: getinfo@haworthpressinc.com].

The HEW Task Force
on Prescription Drugs:
An Insider's Perspective

T. Donald Rucker

INTRODUCTION

In May of 1967, upon a directive from President Lyndon B. Johnson, the Secretary of Health and Human Services (then the U.S. Department of Health, Education and Welfare) established the Task Force on Prescription Drugs. This body was charged with undertaking "a comprehensive study of the problems of including the cost of prescription drugs under Medicare." The Task Force (TF) consisted of nine top officials in the department, including its chairman, Philip R. Lee, M.D., Assistant Secretary for Health, and Staff Director, Milton Silverman, Ph.D. Field work was supported by a professional staff of ten, although effective manpower was probably closer to six full-time equivalents.

During the subsequent months, the TF met periodically to review the work of its staff and to approve the release of the final report and the five background papers that are enumerated in Table I. These

T. Donald Rucker, Ph.D., is Professor of Pharmacy Administration at the College of Pharmacy, University of Illinois at Chicago, M/C 871, Chicago, IL 60612.

Editor's Note: Dr. Rucker can now be reached at 7016 Upland Ridge Drive, Adamstown, MD 21710.

This article was originally published in *Journal of Research in Pharmaceutical Economics*, Vol. 1, No. 1. © The Haworth Press, Inc., 1989.

[Haworth co-indexing entry note]: "The HEW Task Force on Prescription Drugs: An Insider's Perspective." Rucker, T. Donald. Co-published simultaneously in *Journal of Research in Pharmaceutical Economics* (Pharmaceutical Products Press, an imprint of The Haworth Press, Inc.) Vol. 10, No. 2/3, 2001, pp. 5-25; and: *Prescription Drugs Under Medicare: The Legacy of the Task Force on Prescription Drugs* (ed: Mickey C. Smith) Pharmaceutical Products Press, an imprint of The Haworth Press, Inc., 2001, pp. 5-25.

volumes, prepared by Dr. Silverman, total 667 pages and represent a singular achievement both as a conceptual effort and as an accomplishment within the federal bureaucracy.

In addition to developing unique data and extensive surveys of the literature, the staff consulted with various federal agencies and more than 160 representatives from industry, the health professions, academia, consumer groups and foreign governments. Although the project was scheduled for completion in six months, these factors helped to extend the duration to twenty.

In 1968, government (federal and state) outlays for drug benefits under Medicaid (Title 19) amounted to $208 million but had jumped to nearly $3 billion by 1987. With the passage and signing of the Catastrophic Health Insurance Amendments of 1988, which include a prescription drug benefit for aged and disabled individuals protected by Part B of Title 18, these expenditures seem destined to double by 1993 when the law becomes fully operative. Thus basic public policy questions regarding prescription coverage for ambulatory patients have become economically important. This occasion provides, therefore, an opportunity not only to review a pioneering work 20 years later but also to contemplate its value in light of the current legislative reality for which the TF was created.

This critique has been prepared by a health economist who, in 1966, had begun to examine the question of drug insurance for the Social

TABLE I. Publications* of the HEW⁺ Task Force on Prescription Drugs, 1968-1969.

Final Report: Task Force on Prescription Drugs. Washington: GPO, (1969). 86 pages.

Approaches to Drug Insurance Design. Washington: GPO, (1969). 95 pages.

Current American and Foreign Programs. Washington: GPO, (1968). 205 pages.

The Drug Makers and The Drug Distributors. Washington: GPO, (1968). 86 pages.

The Drug Prescribers. Washington: GPO, (1968). 50 pages.

The Drug Users. Washington: GPO, (1968). 145 pages.

---

*Five interim reports were also issued between March 7, 1968, and January 10, 1969, and served, in part, as the basis for the *Final Report*. In light of the substantial documentation furnished in the five background papers, the reason for publication of these reports is unclear.

⁺Since 1980, the U.S. Department of Health and Human Services.

Security Administration and was detailed to aid in the formal investigation; hence the appellation "insider."

RESEARCH, FINDINGS AND RECOMMENDATIONS

As Table II indicates, the call for a comprehensive study of the problems associated with prescription drug benefits led the TF to examine many related issues as well. Consequently, a total of 48 findings and 25 recommendations was put forward. These pertained to drug coverage, the quality of care associated with prescribed medications, the economic use of resources, professional education and proficiency, regulatory considerations at the federal and state level, and federal policy pertaining to pharmaceuticals in general. In short, the TF recognized that optimal drug benefit design could not be realized within the context of the insurance model and that analysis of the complex infrastructure underlying the role of prescribed medications in our society was also necessary.[1]

Drug Benefits for the Aged

The TF reported that many persons 65 years of age and older lacked financial resources to pay for prescribed medicines. Therefore, a need existed for an out-of-hospital insurance program under Medicare.[2] Moreover, such a program "has been shown to be economically feasible in many countries," although "no single method will by itself guarantee program efficiency, but without at least two features–reasonable formulary restrictions and effective data processing procedures–program controls will be ineffective."

In order to ensure reasonable program cost, the TF noted a positive relationship associated with additional features such as copayment or coinsurance (which was preferred over a deductible), use of low-cost chemical equivalents where possible, broad population coverage (to minimize adverse selection), vendor payment based on actual acquisition cost, and drug utilization review (to minimize irrational prescribing). Because of the nascent status of the latter, the TF reported that "there is an urgent need for further research to develop and test various approaches to effective utilization review" as well as a universal coding and classification scheme covering all drug products. For administrative (and probably cost) reasons, the TF stressed that the program provide partial benefits initially, such as those deemed essential in the treatment

TABLE II. Statistical Summary of Task Force Findings and Recommendations According to Primary Area of Inquiry.

Area*	Findings+	Recommendations+
Drug Insurance Benefits for the Aged	1, 2, 6, 9, 10, 12, 17, 20, 21, 22, 24, 26, 27, 28, 29, 30, 31, 32, 33, 34, 35, 36, 37, 38, 39, 40, 41, 42	2(d); 17
Quality of Care: Drug Use Process	8, 11, 14, 18, 19, 21, 28	4, 10, 12, 18(a), (b), (c); 20
Economic Issues	3, 4, 5, 7, 17, 22, 23	1, 2(a), (c), (d); 3(a), (b), (c); 5, 6, 12
Professional Education and Proficiency	8	7(a), (b), (c); 9, 11
HEW/State Government Regulatory Implications	14, 15, 16, 25	2(b); 8, 14, 15, 16, 21, 23, 24, 25
Federal Policy–Pharmaceuticals	13, 16, 43, 44, 45, 46, 47, 48	3(a), (b), (c); 13, 19, 22

* The TF utilized 17 categories for summarizing its work but the six-part framework here provides a more meaningful focus for this critique.

+ As appropriate, several items have been assigned dual classifications.

Source: Task Force on Prescription Drugs. *Final Report.* Washington: GPO, (1969).

of serious long-term illness (i.e., "maintenance drugs"). Finally, physician ownership of repackaging companies was cited as a conflict-of-interest situation that should be prohibited, and the need to study physician dispensing, for the same reason, was noted.

Although some 28 findings pertaining to a drug benefit for ambulatory patients under Medicare were put forward, the TF failed to make a formal recommendation to this effect. Only the transmittal letter from Dr. Lee to the Secretary specified "that such a program be instituted." However, the TF did recommend that more effective methods be found to determine the actual acquisition cost of pharmaceutical products (AWP was recognized as inconsistent with the fiduciary responsibility of a government program), and, further, that several departments test the proposed drug classification system as set forth in Chapter 7: *Approaches to Drug Insurance Design.*

Quality of Care: Drug Use Process

The TF found that prescriber decisions were often suboptimal and believed that cooperation among health professionals, suppliers and government could contribute to more rational prescribing. In addition, it clarified the distinctions between chemical, biological and clinical equivalents and reported that "lack of clinical equivalency among chemical equivalents meeting all official standards has been grossly exaggerated. . . . " Moreover, the TF enumerated certain criteria for implementing a sound formulary while noting that the exclusion of "certain combination products, duplicative drugs, and noncritical products from federal reimbursement would contribute significantly" to both rational prescribing and reduced program cost.

Economic Issues

The TF observed that much of the drug industry's research and development activities appeared "to provide only minor contributions to medical progress." The economic sequelae associated with this result include a waste of skilled resources and a confusing proliferation of drug products that combined to produce a burden on patients or taxpayers who ultimately must pay the costs. Further, the exceptionally high rate of profits attained by large manufacturers was not accompanied by excessive risk or the inability to attract capital.

While the TF was unable to document the efficiency of vendor (pharmacy) operations, it contended that significant program savings must be realized at this level as well. It also contended that payments should be limited to expenses that are directly related to dispensing, and "no portion of program payments should be made for unrelated functions or grossly inefficient vendor services."

Use of low-cost chemical equivalents, when of high quality, could yield savings of approximately five percent at the retail level. Finally, cooperative efforts on the part of professional associations and consumer groups are needed to help patients obtain better information on local prescription prices.

In order to confront these economic issues, the TF recommended that HEW conduct continuing surveys of product costs, prescription prices, and drug use. With respect to the manufacturing industry, it advocated study of incentives to stimulate the discovery and production of significant therapeutic agents and to discourage the output of marginal items. The TF also noted the need to limit the supply of free samples for physicians and to develop more effective methods for ascertaining the actual acquisition costs of prescription products. It called for an interagency investigation to consider discriminatory product pricing practices, discrepancy between foreign and domestic prices for the same product offered by a given firm, and possible revision of patent and trademark laws.

The TF also recommended wider use of prepackaging at the dispensing level, support for research to improve the efficiency and effectiveness of community and hospital pharmacy operations, and publication and distribution of a compendium covering all marketed products with their respective prices.

Professional Education/Proficiency

The inability of most physicians to question their competency in making therapeutic judgments was lamented by the TF. It recommended development of curricula in medical and pharmacy schools to train pharmacists as drug information specialists on the health team. It stressed the desirability of strengthening pharmacy education along with preparation of pharmacy aides to provide their professional superiors with more time to engage in clinical functions. HEW should strengthen the teaching of clinical pharmacology in medical schools and support continuing education for physicians regarding rational prescribing.

Government Regulatory Duties

In reviewing the role of government as a regulator of pharmaceutical products, the TF found that the lack of clinical equivalency among chemical equivalents had been grossly exaggerated. Since uniform standards of product quality and efficacy should apply to all federally-supported drug programs, the committee held that cost differentials due simply to the use of brand or generic terms could not be justified under reimbursement policy. The TF anticipated that the drug efficacy studies of products marketed between 1938 and 1962 would be completed by 1971. It noted that any increase in financial resources required to strengthen controls on product quality should not be attributed to the expense of federally assisted drug programs because these activities benefit the public in general.

The TF recommended that all products licensed for distribution in interstate commerce be subject to the quality control standards established by the FDA and that this agency be provided with adequate financial resources to command internal and external expertise to exercise its scientific and regulatory responsibilities. In addition, it recommended that the FDA establish intramural clinical and laboratory research capabilities to help attract and retain the best scientific personnel. It also specified the need to study whether three classifications–new drugs and "not new" drugs, certifiable products, and biologics–were appropriate to ensure uniform quality. Finally, the TF recommended that HEW support studies on pharmacist licensure and reciprocity to facilitate expanded functions for these professionals and to ensure, rather than impede, fair competition.

Federal Policy

The TF found that a permanent mechanism is needed at the federal level to collect, analyze and exchange information and to provide effective coordination of drug-related activities, such as uniform standards of quality, among the agencies involved. However, it found no need to centralize all drug-related functions within the department. As a result, the regulatory, discovery, manpower, and scientific information divisions of HEW would remain largely as organized.

As reported under the heading "Economic Issues" above, the TF recommended a joint study by the Departments of HEW, Commerce, Justice and other agencies, including the Federal Trade Commission, to consider (1) drug product price differentials that persist between community and hospital pharmacies as well as foreign and domestic suppliers, and (2) the possible revision of patent and trademark laws governing pharmaceutical preparations. One of the major reasons for convening an industry conference was to permit drug firms to specify various marketing practices that could be defined as "unfair trade." These activities would be outlawed and hence place no firm at a competitive disadvantage.

The TF recommended establishment of a Federal Interdepartmental Health Policy Council to coordinate all federal prescription drug purchase and reimbursement programs. It also recommended adoption of a standardized drug code (to facilitate efficiency in processing prescription drug claims) and surveillance of drug costs, prescription prices and drug use by SSA.[3]

AN INDEPENDENT ASSESSMENT

As the *Final Report* of the TF was being issued, a new administration took office in Washington. On March 24, 1969, Secretary Robert H. Finch asked a diverse group of 17 leaders from outside the government to assist him in determining the course of action regarding selected aspects of the Task Force's work.

Within a period of four months, and without staff support, Dr. John T. Dunlop, Professor of Political Economy at Harvard, had elicited a response from each of his Review Committee members covering four basic questions: (1) the feasibility of adding prescription drug coverage to Medicare, (2) federal policy pertaining to chemical/biological/clinical equivalency, (3) economic matters related to drug manufacturing and distribution, and (4) methods for improving the flow of information regarding drugs to practicing physicians.

With only one dissent, the Review Committee concluded that the Medicare program should be expanded to include drug benefits and that HEW should develop more detailed plans concerning program regulations, data processing procedures, and cost computations necessary for legislative consideration. However, the Committee noted that (1) limitation of benefits to chronic disease treatments was neither advisable nor administrable, (2) an age limitation above 65 was undesirable, (3) a deductible should be avoided because of the record-keeping burden it placed on patients, (4) that copayment was preferable to coinsurance, and (5) only a "purely advisory national formulary . . . might possibly be appropriate." The drug program should be built around copayment (with perhaps an annual ceiling beyond which the patient could be reimbursed), vendor payment based on a flat dispensing fee, coverage under Part A, and utilization review.

In discussing the pharmacologic issues, the Committee recommended that the FDA continue developing reference standards for generic drugs to assure biologic equivalency, that advisory committees be established to assist in evaluating compliance with such standards, and that improved quality control in drug manufacturing through registration/licensure, as called for by the TF, be supported.

When the Review Committee confronted the major economic questions, there was general agreement that (1) pharmaceutical manufacturers' profits are high, relative to other industries; (2) a study should be made of price differentials that exist when products are sold to various types of buyers; and (3) patients need better information about prescription prices. The Committee recommended that the department support research to improve the efficiency of community and hospital pharmacy operations and generally prohibit reimbursement of physician-owned repackaging companies. However, there was less agreement among Committee members regarding the TF finding concerning duplicate and wasteful research by drug manufacturers.

With respect to TF recommendations pertaining to better information for prescribers, the Review Committee supported guidelines concerned with rational drug therapy and publication of a comprehensive compendium. In both cases though, it contended that the scientific basis for these compilations should emanate from nongovernment sources, although major funding would be supplied by the public purse.

Given the fact that eight of the Committee members were provider-oriented, the extent of consensus regarding government policy on prescription drugs seems nothing less than remarkable.

IMPACT OF THE TASK FORCE'S WORK

The impact of the Task Force on Prescription Drugs is difficult to assess because results are a function of different criteria that may be employed and of evaluator interpretation. With respect to legislative efforts to extend drug coverage for aged persons, numerous bills were introduced in the Congress for many years after the *Final Report* was issued in February 1969. However, during the 3-4 years prior to that date, more than 50 bills were introduced. While comparison of legislative components might be attempted via content analysis, the TF never recommended a model law as such. In fact, no administration–Republican or Democratic–has ever sponsored a bill to add prescription benefits to Medicare or even included them in a national health insurance plan. If the drug benefit under the 1988 amendments is used for analysis, the major staff paper[4] shaping this legislation incorporated only one reference (out of 71) that might be traced to the TF effort.

The impact of the TF may also be inferred from the literature dealing with drug insurance and related issues as outlined in Table II. In this connection, the selected references presented in the Appendix reflect a major extension of the drug policy and drug insurance activities initiated by the TF. The prolific output of Dr. Silverman and associates represents a significant achievement in delineating major policy issues on the domestic scene and affecting changes in promotional and information practices conducted by large multinational pharmaceutical firms within many developing nations. A uniform cost accounting system for community pharmacy, developed by Dr. Bruce R. Siecker, stands as a beacon that illuminates how economic data should serve as the cornerstone for determining vendor reimbursement.

Studies such as those by Avorn,[5] Ray,[6] Richards,[7] and Soumerai,[8] coupled with important publications by USP[9,10,11] and AMA,[12] treat various aspects of the central questions addressed by the TF. However, neither of the compendia published by USP and AMA incorporates the product price information so strongly advocated by the TF. While methods of introducing price information into clinical decision making represent a complex topic beyond the focus of this overview, adding price data to compendia raises questions about relative effectiveness of alternative models: (1) should not the physician give first consideration to selecting the drug of choice; (2) should not physicians have access to all prices per therapeutic category via computer terminal, rather than a published document, when they are originating a prescription order; and (3) should not reimbursement policy constitute the primary foundation for adjudicating product prices rather than trying to transform a busy clinician into a haphazard drug economist?[13]

If one moves from the legislative and literature models to the impact that the TF had on bureaucratic function, one can claim that its work stimulated FDA to establish external advisory panels of outside experts to review New Drug Applications and develop the National Drug Code Directory. Unfortunately, the efficiency of this universal coding system was vitiated when the Pharmaceutical Manufacturers Association insisted that each multiple source product be identified by both a manufacturer's prefix and a unique 4-digit code.

The TF was also instrumental in inducing FDA (via NAS/NRI) to review the efficacy of drugs approved between 1938 and 1962 (DESI project). In 1987, though, the Health Care Financing Administration was still listing 107 drug products identified by the DESI program as ineligible for reimbursement under Medicaid.[14] The TF recommendation for transferring the Division of Biologic Standards from NIH to

FDA was carried out. Finally, the TF facilitated the agency's role "in dealing with the complex problems of drug quality, chemical equivalents, bioavailability, and clinical equivalency."[15]

DISCUSSION

The work of the TF represented the first systematic attempt by the administrative branch of the federal government to define and evaluate major public policy issues associated with drug use and insurance beyond the traditional regulatory matters pertaining to product purity, safety and efficacy. In this endeavor, the TF made available the first national profile of drug use among the elderly; defined rational prescribing; documented the prevalence of irrational prescribing; and stressed the contribution that drug utilization review[16] could make, first in reducing inappropriate prescribing, and secondly in controlling program cost. The TF also put forward a number of innovative proposals, such as the idea that exclusive rights to a product's trademark should last no longer than the patent, that drug program design should be simple enough that patients do not become unduly burdened in obtaining benefits and that drug programs under Medicare and Medicaid should be coordinated.

The TF disclosed the nature of drug industry profits and resources dissipated in the marketing of products. It also demonstrated the waste associated with most "me-too" products and fixed combination preparations. It emphasized the potential value of clinical pharmacists' contributions to program goals and patient health status.

While many of these issues have subsequently entered the public domain, some were sufficiently radical to induce the President of PMA to make a personal trip to HEW in the spring of 1972 to help derail the research of the Drug Studies Branch in the Department[17] that focused on his clients. While the TF contributions to social welfare were numerous, the Committee also waffled, calling for more study of the role of physician-owned pharmacies, dispensing physicians, and, understandably, methods an insurance program should follow to reimburse providers for product cost. In addition, the *Final Report* was so preoccupied with identifying competing formula for reimbursing vendors for product cost and professional overhead that it neglected to mention what type of data was required for closely approximating the true economic cost of an efficient provider, regardless of methodology.

The TF pointed out the financial reasons for adding drug benefits to Part A of Medicare, but it never recognized the value of merging physician and drug claims under Part B as a means of making the DUR function more effectively. Further, while stressing the patient burden of records-keeping associated with a high deductible, the *Final Report* did not point out that this means of patient cost-sharing is also likely to decimate quality assurance activities designed to raise beneficiary health status.

Although the TF provided a clear statement regarding the contribution of a drug formulary to program administration, it probably distorted our understanding of this mechanism by failing to differentiate between limitations in the scope of benefits (deletion of an entire therapeutic category) and formulary restrictions within an approved category. It also failed to clarify that administrative controls on drug quantity and product price can be promulgated in the absence of a formulary and hence such measures should not be ascribed to formulary performance for either positive or negative attribution.

The TF confused the reason for providing drug benefits only to patients who had reached age 70 or 72 (all retirement and Medicare benefits commence when an individual reaches age 65). Because cost, both initially and subsequently, is always a consideration with any federal program, the argument was advanced that a higher age limit was one means of dealing with the cost constraint. However, this proposal was suggested by staff to confront the claim volume problem with the understanding that the age limit would be temporary and dropped to 65 just as soon as claim processing capabilities permitted rapid handling of the larger administrative load.

The department never tested the drug classification system discussed above, but the Veterans Administration has utilized this source in preparing its own system.[18] Finally, the problem of inappropriate prescribing and inadequate education for prescribers remains[19] despite the heroic efforts of the TF to confront this social malady. Perhaps the 1988 addition of drug benefits to the Medicare program will help resurrect this and other public policy matters initiated by the HEW Task Force on Prescription Drugs two decades ago.

POSTSCRIPT

Two incidents related to the work of the TF illustrate a basic social problem concerning the relationship of the pharmaceutical manufacturing industry to efforts to develop prudent public policy.

During the latter part of 1968, an attorney employed by one of the largest drug firms approached the author for an advance copy of the *Third* or *Fourth Interim Report*. When he perceived after several minutes of discussion that I was unwilling to provide this document (it was sitting in a filing cabinet less than a foot from his head), he snorted, "Oh, the hell with it, we will steal it," and stomped out of the room.

The second incident occurred a decade later when the author was a professor in Columbus, Ohio. A representative from another large firm stopped for an unannounced visit as had often been his practice during my seven-year tenure in Washington. It was now a rare event, however, for him, or any other industry official, to make the trek to the Midwest for business or social purposes.

"Well, Alan, what are you doing in town?" I asked. "Oh," he remarked, "headquarters wants to know what our pricing policy is and I am doing a field survey among our customers to find out what they paid for our products!" A decade later, another official of the same firm appeared in my office in Chicago. When I related this incident about his employer, he responded, "I can understand that."

These two examples illustrate how arrogance and obfuscation often stand as impediments to the development of a reimbursement policy that attempts to encompass the legitimate claims of both providers and society.

REFERENCES

1. Given the provisions of drug coverage under the Medicare Catastrophic Health Insurance Amendments of 1988, it seems impossible that a similar claim could be made for the current legislation.

2. In the early 1970s, Medicare coverage was expanded to include several million disabled persons and their dependents who qualified for monthly benefits under Social Security. This group has a utilization rate for prescribed drugs that exceeds that of aged individuals.

3. A similar recommendation today would assign this duty to HCFA.

4. Office of Technology Assessment. *Prescription drugs and elderly Americans: ambulatory use and approaches to coverage for Medicare*. Washington: U.S. Congress, (October 1987); 68 pages.

5. Avorn, J. & Soumerai, S.B. Improving drug-therapy decisions through educational outreach: a randomized controlled trial of academically based "detailing." *New England Journal of Medicine*, 308 (June 16, 1983); 1457-63.

6. Ray, W.A., Schaffner, W., & Federspiel, C.F. Persistence of improvement in antibiotic prescribing in office practice. *Journal of the American Medical Association*, 253 (March 22/29, 1985): 1774-76.

7. Richards, J.W. Third party prescription programs: cost containment issues and strategies. *American Pharmacy*, NS25 (July 1985): 28-35.

8. Soumerai, S.B., Avorn, J., et al. Payment restrictions for prescription drugs under Medicaid. *New England Journal of Medicine*, 317 (August 27, 1987): 550-56.

9. USP. *Guide to select drugs*. Rockville, MD: United States Pharmacopoeial Convention, (1975).

10. USP. *USP DI–Drug information for the health care professional*, (2 vol.). Rockville, MD: United States Pharmacopoeial Convention, (1988).

11. USP. *USP DI–Advice for the Patient*. Rockville, MD: United States Pharmacopoeial Convention, (1988).

12. AMA Division of Drugs. *AMA drug evaluations*, (5th ed.). Chicago: American Medical Association, (1983).

13. Rucker, T.D. Commentary on: A.M. Lee, Constraining costs on pharmaceutical programs: lessons from abroad. In: *Impact of Public Policy on Drug Innovation and Pricing*, Mitchell, S.A. & Link, E.A. (eds.). Washington: The American University, (1976); 188.

14. Anon. HCFA guide to DESI drugs. *Drug Store News–Inside Pharmacy*, 9 (April 1987): 31-37.

15. Lee, P.R. The task force on prescription drugs. *Drug Information Journal*, 11 (January/March, 1977): 7-10.

16. The TF emphasized that DUR represented a continuing process of claim evaluation and noted how this function differed from the traditional one of claim administration. The concept may be confusing to some because in recent years investigators have employed various handles, such as drug use evaluation and drug usage review, to discuss the basic quality assurance process. The TF, however, failed to admonish us that the major objective of DUR is to go out of business, i.e., to become so successful in the retrospective mode that review procedures would be incorporated in clinical decision making and patient treatment. Finally, DUR effectiveness may be jeopardized to the extent that inept politicians and zealous administrators depend upon this educational process to offset deficiencies in reimbursement policy.

17. *The Washington Post*. (April 28, 1972).

18. USP. *USP DI–Drug information for the health care professional*, (Vol. II). Rockville, MD: United States Pharmacopoeial Convention, (1988): Appendix III.

19. Health and Policy Committee, American College of Physicians. Improving medical education in therapeutics. *Annals of Internal Medicine*, 108 (January 1988): 147-47.

APPENDIX

Selected References Prompted
by the Work of the Task Force
on Prescription Drugs

American Pharmaceutical Association. *White paper on the pharmacist's role in product selection.* Washington: APhA, (1971).

Berger, B.A. Coverage of non-drug items under a major drug insurance program. *Pharmacy Management,* 152 (May-June 1980): 110-112;117.

Brodie, R.C. *Drug utilization and drug utilization review and control.* Health Services and Mental Health Administration. DHEW Pub. No. (HSM) 72-3002, (1970).

Campbell, W.H., Johnson, R.E. & Christensen, D.B. A procedural and conceptual analysis of drug use review. *Drugs in Health Care,* 2 (Fall 1975): 211-30.

Christensen, D.B. Guiding principles for pharmacy services under national health insurance. *Pharmacy Management,* 152 (September-October 1980): 205-09.

Cotton, H.A. & Rucker, T.D. Prescription cost determination in Kansas. *Journal American Pharmaceutical Association,* NS12 (August 1972): 412-15.

Fink, J.L. Some legal aspects of the hospital formulary system. *American Journal of Hospital Pharmacy,* 31 (January 1974): 86-90.

Fink, J.L. Coverage of prescription drugs for non-hospitalized Medicare patients. *Clearinghouse Law Review,* 8 (February 1975): 712-20.

Fink, J.L. *Manager's guide to third-party programs.* Washington: American Pharmaceutical Association, (1982); 90 pages.

Fulda, T.R. Drug cost control: the road to maximum allowable cost regulations. In: *Toward a national health policy, public policy in the control of health care cost,* Freidman, K. & Raxoff, S., (eds.). Lexington, MA: Lexington Books, (1977); 55-67.

Gagnon, J.P., et al. A comparison of maintenance and nonmaintenance outpatient prescription directions, duration of coverage and costs per day. *Medical Care,* 13 (January 1975): 47-58.

Gagnon, J.P. & Rodowskas, C.A. Two controversial problems in third-party outpatient prescription plans. *Journal of Risk and Insurance,* 39 (December 1972): 603-11.

Gardner, V. Maximum allowable cost: estimated acquisition cost. *California Pharmacist,* 24 (July 1976): 36-39.

Health Care Financing Administration. *Guide to prescription drug costs.* Baltimore: HCFA-02104, (April 1980).

Jacoby, E.M. & Hefner, D.L. Domestic and foreign prescription drug prices. *Social Security Bulletin*, 34 (May 1971): 15-22.

Johnson, R.C. Overview and objectives of drug program management. *California Pharmacist*, 25 (January 1978): 19-24.

Knapp, D.A. & Palumbo, F.B. *Containing costs in third party programs.* Hamilton, IL: Drug Intelligence Publications, Inc., (1978).

Knapp, D.A. Review article: paying for outpatient prescription drugs and related services in third party programs. *Medical Care Review*, 28 (August 1971): 826-59.

Knapp, D.A. The restrictive formulary and drug use review in a Medicare out-of-hospital prescription drug program. *NARD Journal*, 95 (October 15, 1973): 14-16.

Lee, P.R. The task force on prescription drugs: a review of problems, progress and possibilities. *Drug Information Journal*, 11 (March 1977): 7-10.

Lipton, H.L. & Lee, P.R. *Drugs and the elderly.* Stanford, CA: Stanford Univ. Press, (1988).

Maronde, R.F., et al. A study of prescribing patterns. *Medical Care*, 9 (September/October 1971); 383-95.

Maronde, R.F., et al. Drug data processing: its role in the control of drug abuse. *California Medicine*, 117 (September 1972): 22-28.

Maronde, R.F. & Silverman, M. Prescribing hypnotic and anti-anxiety drugs. *Annals Internal Medicine*, 79 (September 1973):452.

Maronde, R.F. *Drug utilization review with on-line computer capability.* ORS/SSA, staff paper #13, DHEW Pub. No. (SSA) 73-11853, (1972); 81 pages.

Maronde, R.F. Drug utilization review. In: *Perspectives on medicines in society*, Wertheimer, A.I. & Bush, P.J. (eds.). Hamilton, IL: Drug intelligence Publications, (1977); 169-91.

Massachusetts Department of Public Health. The Massachusetts drug formulary. *New England Journal Medicine*, 285 (July 22, 1971): 232-33.

Morse, M.L., et al. Reducing drug therapy-induced hospitalization: impact of drug utilization review. *Drug Information Journal*, 16 (October/December 1982): 199-202.

Muller, C. Drug benefits in health insurance. *International Journal Health Services*, 4 (Winter 1974): 157-70.

Muller, C. Payment mechanisms. In: *Perspectives on medicines in society*, Wertheimer, A.I. & Bush, P.J. (eds.). Hamilton, IL: Drug Intelligence Publications; 429-49, (1977).

Olejar, P.D. (ed.). *Proceedings: computer-based information system in the practice of pharmacy.* Chapel Hill, NC: School of Pharmacy, University of North Carolina, (1971); 199 pages.

Pan American Health Organization. *Development and implementation of drug formularies.* Washington: PAHO Scientific Publication 474, (1984).

Report of the Secretary's Review Committee of the Task Force on Prescription Drugs, (T. Dunlop, chairman). Washington: Office of the Secretary, U.S. Dept. HEW, (July 23,1969); 164 pages.

Rucker, T.D. Pharmacy and third parties in the 1970's. *Michigan Pharmacist,* 7 (July 1970): 829-34.

Rucker, T.D. The need for drug utilization review. *American Journal Hospital Pharmacy,* 27 (August 1970): 654-58.

Rucker, T.D. Drug insurance and vendor compensation. *California Pharmacist,* 18 (October 1970): 20-27.

Rucker, T.D. Possible impact of a government drug program on community pharmacies. *Journal American Pharmaceutical Association,* NS11 (June 1971): 334-37.

Rucker, T.D. Problems in measuring overhead costs for prescription services. *Texas Pharmacy,* 90 (October 1971): 24-37.

Rucker, T.D. Drug insurance, formularies and pharmacy. *Medical Marketing & Media,* 6 (October 1971): 11-18.

Rucker, T.D. The role of computers in drug utilization review. *American Journal Hospital Pharmacy,* 29 (February 1972): 128-33.

Rucker, T.D. The pharmacist and national health insurance–potentials and problems. *California Pharmacist,* 19 (April 1972): 24-29.

Rucker, T.D. Economic problems in drug distribution. *Inquiry,* 9 (September 1972): 43-50.

Rucker, T.D. A model information system for prescription drug services. *Wisconsin Pharmacist,* 41 (December 1972): 411-15.

Rucker, T.D. National health insurance–prerequisites and principles. *Wisconsin Pharmacist,* 42 (January 1973): 33-38.

Rucker, T.D. Theory and practice in drug insurance design. *Illinois Pharmacist,* 37 (January 1973): 25-29.

Rucker, T.D. Economic aspects of drug overuse. *Medical Annals of the District of Columbia,* 42 (December 1973): 609-14.

Rucker, T.D. & Krautheim, D. A computer-oriented pharmacy information system: macro considerations. *Journal of Clinical Computing,* 3 (January 1974): 317-28.

Rucker, T.D. Public policy considerations in the use of psychoactive drugs. *Drugs in Health Care,* 1 (Summer 1974): 5-15.

Rucker, T.D. Public policy considerations in the pricing of prescription drugs. *International Journal Health Services,* 4 (Winter 1974): 171-79.

Rucker, T.D. The pharmaceutical manufacturing industry's role in a dynamic health care system. *Drugs in Health Care,* 2 (Spring 1975): 86-95.

Rucker, T.D. Drug information for prescribers and dispensers: toward a model system. *Medical Care*, 14 (February 1976): 156-65.

Rucker, T.D. Commentary on: A.M. Lee, Constraining costs on pharmaceutical programs: lessons from abroad. In: *Impact of public policy on drug innovation and pricing*, Mitchell, S.A. & Link, E.A. (eds.). Washington: The American University, (1976); 177-89.

Rucker, T.D. Commentary on: Gordon Trapnell, Medicaid drug insurance progress: a comparison of the effect of contrasting approaches. In: *Impact of public policy on drug innovation and pricing*, Mitchell, S.A. & Link, E.A. (eds.). Washington: The American University, (1976); 230-33.

Rucker, T.D. National health insurance and prescription benefits. *Drug Intelligence & Clinical Pharmacy*, 10 (September 1976): 529-33.

Rucker, T.D. Around and beyond UCAS: the road to economic survival for community pharmacy. *Journal American Pharmaceutical Association*, NS17 (May 1977): 292-96.

Rucker, T.D. How to survive in a sea of government programs. *American Journal of Pharmacy*, 149 (July-August 1977): 106-12.

Rucker, T.D. Reimbursement policy under drug insurance: administrative expediency or economic validity? *American Journal of Pharmacy*, 150 (July/August 1978): 107-18.

Rucker, T.D., Janis, L. & Bennett, M. Prescriptions ordered by podiatrists for ambulatory patients: an exploratory study. *Drug Intelligence & Clinical Pharmacy*, 12 (December 1978): 720-27.

Rucker, T.D. Third party drug programs: an overview. *Pharmacy Management*, 151 (January 1979): 26-28.

Rucker, T.D. & Visconti, J.A. *How effective are drug formularies? A descriptive and normative study*. Washington: American Society of Hospital Pharmacists Research & Education Foundation, (1979).

Rucker, T.D. Prescription drug coverage: insurance or prepayment? *Pharmacy Management*, 151 (July/August 1979): 171-73.

Rucker, T.D. & Visconti, J.A. Relative drug safety & efficacy: any help for the practitioner? *American Journal Hospital Pharmacy*, 36 (August 1979): 1099-1101.

Rucker, T.D. & Grover, R.A. Coverage of OTC preparations under prepayment programs. *Pharmacy Management*, 151 (November/December 1979): 254-57.

Rucker, T.D. Prescription drug benefits under national health insurance–a blue ribbon proposal. *Pharmacy Management*, 152 (January/February 1980): 23-28.

Rucker, T.D. The top-selling drug products: how good are they? *American Journal Hospital Pharmacy*, 37 (June 1980): 833-37.

Rucker, T.D. & Morse, M.L. The Medicaid drug program in Louisiana:

critique of the Hefner-Pracon study. *American Journal Hospital Pharmacy*, 37 (October 1980): 1350-53; 38 (March 1981): 304.

Rucker, T.D. Effective formulary development: which direction? *Topics in Hospital Pharmacy Management*, 1 (May 1981): 29-45.

Rucker, T.D., Duche, G., & Clasen, T.E. Clinical pharmacy: a strategy for community practitioners. *Contemporary Pharmacy Practice*, 5 (Winter 1982): 21-26.

Rucker, T.D. Prescription drug insurance: a traditional or trustee role? *Pharmacy International*, 3 (June 1982): 196-98.

Rucker, T.D. Formularies: conceptual and experiential factors related to drug product selection. *Drug Information Journal*, 16 (July/September 1982): 115-21.

Rucker, T.D. Superior hospital formularies: a critical analysis. *Hospital Pharmacy*, 17 (September 1982): 465-524.

Rucker, T.D. Drug utilization review: moving toward an effective safe model. In: *Society and medication: conflicting signals for prescribers and patients*, Morgan, J.P. & Kagan, D.V., (eds.). Lexington, MA: Lexington Books, D.C. Heath & Co., (1983); 25-51.

Rucker, T.D. Selected problems in drug nomenclature. *Journal of Clinical Computing*, 12(1/2) (1983): 31-34.

Rucker, T.D. Putting reimbursement policy back on the track. *Hospital Pharmacy*, 18 (August 1983): 404-05.

Rucker, T.D. Computerization of prescription data with particular reference to drug nomenclature. *Journal of Clinical Computing*, 13(2/3) (1984): 28-34.

Rucker, T.D. Micro/Macro strategies for improving hospital formulary performance. *Clinical Research Practice Drug Regulatory Affairs*, 2(3) (1984): 295-312.

Rucker, T. D. The role of formularies and their relationship to drug product selection. In: *Generic drug laws: a decade of trial–a prescription for progress*, Goldberg, T., Devito, C.A., & Raskin, I.E. (eds.). National Center for Health Services Research, U.S. Dept. HHS, Washington, (June 1986); 465-85.

Rucker, T.D. Prescribed medications: system control or therapeutic roulette? IFAC Monograph: *Control aspects of biomedical engineering*, Nalecz, Maciej, (ed.). Oxford, England: Pergamon Press, (1987); 167-75.

Rucker, T.D. Pursuing rational drug therapy: a macro view a la the USA. *Journal Social Administrative Pharmacy*, 5(3) (1988): 76-85.

Schifrin, L.G. Economics and epidemiology of drug use. In: *Clinical Pharmacology*, Melmon, K.L. & Morrelli, H.F. (eds.). New York: Macmillan Pub. Co., (1978); 1084-1109.

Siecker, B.R. Pharmacy economics and principles of uniform cost accounting. *Journal American Pharmaceutical Association,* NS15 (December 1975): 678-82.

Siecker, B.R. The uniform cost accounting approach for pharmacy pricing decisions. *Journal American Pharmaceutical Association,* NS17 (April 1977): 208-12.

Siecker, B.R. *Uniform cost accounting approach for pharmacy–UCAS.* Washington: American Pharmaceutical Association, (1979).

Silverman, M. & Lee, P.R. *Pills, profits and politics.* Berkeley, CA: University of California Press, (1974).

Silverman, M. & Lydecker, M. Prescription drug pricing by hospital pharmacies. *American Journal Hospital Pharmacy,* 31 (September 1974): 870.

Silverman, M. *The drugging of the Americas.* Berkeley, CA: University of California Press, (1976).

Silverman, M. The epidemiology of drug promotion. *International Journal Health Services,* 7(2) (1977): 157.

Silverman, M. & Lydecker, M. *Drug coverage under national health insurance: the policy options.* National Center for Health Services Research, DHEW Pub. No. (HRA) 77-3189, (1977).

Silverman, M. Who needs drug insurance. *Hospital Formulary,* 13 (February 1978): 138.

Silverman, M. & Lydecker, M., (eds.). *Proceedings of the national conference on drug coverage under national health insurance.* National Center for Health Services Research, DHEW Pub. No. (PHS) 78-3208, (1978).

Silverman, M. Pharmacy, society, and upcoming federal legislation. *California Pharmacist,* 27 (October, 1979): 38.

Silverman, M. & Lee, P.R. The revolution in drugs. And, Future strategy: prescriptions for action. In: *The Nation's Health,* Lee, P.R., Brown, N. & Red, I. (eds.). San Francisco: Boyd & Fraser, (1981).

Silverman, M. & Lydecker, M. The promotion of prescription drugs and other puzzles. In: *Pharmaceutical and Health Policy,* Blum, R. et al. (eds.). New York: Holmes & Meier Publishers, (1981).

Silverman, M., Lee, P.R., & Lydecker, M. *Pills & the public purse.* Berkeley, CA: University of California Press, (1981).

Silverman, M., Lee, P.R. & Lydecker, M. *Prescriptions for death: the drugging of the third world.* Berkeley, CA: University of California Press, (1982).

Silverman, M., Lee, P.R. & Lydecker, M. Drug promotion: the third world revisited. *International Journal of Health Services,* 16(4) (1986): 659.

Smith, M.C. & Wilkinson, W.E. Automation of vendor drug claims. *Journal American Pharmaceutical Association,* NS10 (September 1968): 501-05.

Smith, M.C., Mikeal, R.L. & Wilkinson, W.E. Studies in the automation of vendor drug claims. *Journal American Pharmaceutical Association*, NS12 (April 1972): 156-65.

Smith, M.C. Pharmacy and national health insurance. In: *Pharmacy in health care and institutional systems*, Lecca, P.J. & Tharp, C.P. (eds.). St. Louis: C.V. Mosby, (1978); 13-46.

Stolley, P.D. & Goddard, J.L. Prescription drug insurance for the elderly under Medicare. *American Journal Public Health*, 61 (March 1971): 574-81.

Strom, B.L., et al. Drug antisubstitution studies: estimation of possible savings by repeal of antisubstitution laws. *Drugs in Health Care*, 1 (Fall 1974): 99-103.

Wertheimer, A.I. (ed.). *Proceedings of the international conference on drug and pharmaceutical services reimbursement*. National Center for Health Services Research. DHEW Pub. No. (HRA) 77-3186, (1977).

Wolfe, S.M., et al. *Worst pills, best pills*. Washington: Public Citizen Health Research Group, (1988).

Editor's Note

What follows is the Final Report of the Task Force on Prescription Drugs. As noted in Dr. Lee's memorandum to the Secretary of what was then the Department of Health, Education and Welfare, the work of the Task Force took nearly two years. While the report reproduced here is lengthy, it is backed by five equally lengthy background reports:

- The Drug Users
- The Drug Makers and the Drug Distributors
- The Drug Prescribers
- Current American and Foreign Programs
- Approaches to Drug Insurance Design

While the major findings of each are a part of the Final Report reproduced here, each of the background papers is fascinating reading in its own right.

In addition to the obviously important recommendations regarding such things as formularies, clinical equivalency, and the need for a national drug classification system–all of which had far-reaching re-sults–students of history will wish to examine the list of names at the end of the report. Rarely, if ever, has such a representative cross section of interested parties been systematically involved in a drug policy endeavor.

[Haworth co-indexing entry note]: "Editor's Note." Smith, Mickey C. Co-published simultaneously in *Journal of Research in Pharmaceutical Economics* (Pharmaceutical Products Press, an imprint of The Haworth Press, Inc.) Vol. 10, No. 2/3, 2001, p. 27; and: *Prescription Drugs Under Medicare: The Legacy of the Task Force on Prescription Drugs* (ed: Mickey C. Smith) Pharmaceutical Products Press, an imprint of The Haworth Press, Inc., 2001, p. 27. Single or multiple copies of this article are available for a fee from The Haworth Document Delivery Service [1-800-342-9678, 9:00 a.m. - 5:00 p.m. (EST). E-mail address: getinfo@haworthpressinc.com].

Final Report

TASK FORCE ON PRESCRIPTION DRUGS

Philip R. Lee, M.D.
Assistant Secretary for Health
and Scientific Affairs
(Chairman)

Dean Coston
Executive Assistant to the Secretary

James F. Kelly
Assistant Secretary, Comptroller

Alice M. Rivlin, Ph.D.[1]
Assistant Secretary for Planning and
Evaluation

Robert M. Ball
Commissioner, Social Security
Administration

Herbert L. Ley, Jr., M.D.[2]
Commissioner, Food and Drug
Administration

Joseph H. Meyers
Deputy Administrator, Social
and Rehabilitation Service

William H. Stewart, M.D.
Surgeon General, Public Health
Service

Milton Silverman, Ph.D.
Special Assistant to the Assistant
Secretary for Health and Scientific Affairs
*(Executive Secretary and Staff
Director)*

[1]Succeeded William Gorham, on July 1, 1968.
[2]Succeeded James L. Goddard, M.D. on
July 1, 1968.

TASK FORCE STAFF

Mark Novitch, M.D.
(Assistant Staff Director)

Allen J. Brands, R.PH.

Vincent Gardner

Juanita P. Horton, R.PH.

Riley J. Jeansone, R.PH.

Bradley P. Neer, D.V.M.

T. Donald Rucker, Ph.D.

William G. Shoemaker, R.PH.

Vincent E. Vandre

Patricia A. Vienna

Editorial

Alice Haywood

Mia Lydecker

Janeth Page

[Haworth co-indexing entry note]: "Final Report." Task Force on Prescription Drugs. Co-published simultaneously in *Journal of Research in Pharmaceutical Economics* (Pharmaceutical Products Press, an imprint of The Haworth Press, Inc.) Vol. 10, No. 2/3, 2001, pp. 29-180; and: *Prescription Drugs Under Medicare: The Legacy of the Task Force on Prescription Drugs* (ed: Mickey C. Smith) Pharmaceutical Products Press, an imprint of The Haworth Press, Inc., 2001, pp. 29-180. Single or multiple copies of this article are available for a fee from The Haworth Document Delivery Service [1-800-342-9678, 9:00 a.m. - 5:00 p.m. (EST). E-mail address: getinfo@haworthpressinc.com].

UNITED STATES   DEPARTMENT OF HEALTH, EDUCATION,
GOVERNMENT   AND WELFARE
OFFICE OF THE SECRETARY

MEMORANDUM

TO: The Secretary   DATE: February 7, 1969
FROM: Philip R. Lee, M.D. Assistant Secretary for Health and Scientific Affairs
SUBJECT: Task Force on Prescription Drugs–Final Report

In May of 1967, upon a directive from the President, the Task Force on Prescription Drugs was established to undertake a comprehensive study of the problems of including the costs of prescription drugs under Medicare.

During the ensuing 20 months, the Task Force carried out a number of studies involved in this complex assignment. Based on this work, we have already completed and submitted five interim reports.

I am now pleased to transmit for your consideration the final report, which summarizes the major findings and recommendations previously included in the interim reports. Perhaps the most significant are these:

- The finding that a drug insurance program under Medicare is needed by the elderly and would be both economically and medically feasible, and the recommendation that such a program be instituted.

- The finding that the once-confusing matter of clinical equivalency is far less complex than had been anticipated, and that as a result of current laboratory and clinical studies–initiated in large part in response to requests by the Task Force–the problem is well on its way to a solution.

A number of the recommendations submitted by the Task Force have been acted upon by Secretary Gardner and Secretary Cohen. Some of these have involved actions within the Department of Health, Education, and Welfare. Others have involved close and effective cooperation with private organizations and institutions.

Some of the important recommendations have been communicated to all the physicians of the country, as well as to the deans of relevant professional schools and leaders of professional health organizations. Many constructive suggestions have been received as a result of these efforts.

Several recommendations will require legislative action and therefore have not yet been implemented. Still others will require formal agreements among various Federal Departments and agencies; action on these was deferred by Secretary Cohen because of the long-term commitments which would be involved.

In addition to these reports, the Task Force and its staff have prepared a series of background papers on various aspects of the use, production, distribution, and prescription of drugs, and the nature of current drug insurance programs. Four of these volumes–*The Drug Users, The Drug Makers and the Drug Distributors, The Drug Prescribers*, and *Current American and Foreign Programs*–have already been published. A fifth–on approaches to drug insurance design–is now being completed.*

It is our hope that these reports and background publications will be useful as the basis for careful analysis and discussion, and that they will serve as a contribution to the improvement of the quality of health care throughout the Nation.

TERMINOLOGY

The term *generic equivalents* is not used in the body of this report. Although it has been widely utilized, it has been given so many

---

*Editor's note: Each of these is now available.

different interpretations that it has become confusing. Instead, the following terms are used:

Chemical equivalents–Those multiple-source drug products which contain essentially identical amounts of the identical active, ingredients, in identical dosage forms, and which meet existing physicochemical standards in the official compendia.

Biological equivalents–Those chemical equivalents which, when administered in the same amounts, will provide essentially the same biological or physiological availability, as measured by blood levels, etc.

Clinical equivalents–Those chemical equivalents which, when administered in the same amounts, will provide essentially the same therapeutic effect as measured by the control of a symptom or a disease.

The following are terms also used:

Generic name–The *established* or *official* name given to a drug or drug product.

Brand name–The registered trademark name given to a specific drug product by its manufacturer.

Molecular manipulation–A minor modification in the molecular structure of a chemical, yielding a new and patentable product which may or may not offer a significant therapeutic advantage over a related drug already on the market.

"Me-too" or "duplicative" drug–A new drug, often made by means of molecular manipulation, which offers no significant therapeutic advantage over a related drug already on the market. (Chemical equivalents, since they are chemically identical, are not considered to be "me-too" products.)

Rational prescribing–Prescribing the right drug for the right patient, at the right time, in the right amounts, and with due consideration of relative costs.

SUMMARY OF MAJOR FINDINGS

The Drug Users

1. The requirements for appropriate prescription drug therapy by the elderly are very great–far greater, in fact, then those of any other group–and many elderly men and women are now unable

to meet those needs with their limited incomes, savings, or present insurance coverage. Their inability to afford the drugs they require may well be reflected in needless sickness and disability, unemployability, and costly hospitalization which could have been prevented by adequate out-of-hospital treatment.*

2. In order to improve the access of the elderly to high quality health care, and to protect them where possible against high drug expenses which they may be unable to meet, there is need for an out-of-hospital drug insurance program under Medicare.

The Drug Makers

3. Since important new chemical entities represent only a fraction–perhaps 10 to 25 percent–of all new products introduced each year, and the remainder consists merely of minor modifications or combination products, then much of the drug industry's research and development activities would appear to provide only minor contributions to medical progress.

4. To the extent the industry directs a share of its research program to duplicative, noncontributory products, there is a waste of skilled research manpower and research facilities, a waste of clinical facilities needed to test the products, a further confusing proliferation of drug products which are promoted to physicians, and a further burden on the patient or taxpayer who, in the long run, must pay the costs.

5. The exceptionally high rate of profit which generally marks the drug industry is not accompanied by any peculiar degree of risk, or by any unique difficulties in obtaining growth capital. Industry profits have not been significantly reduced by new governmental regulations concerning drug safety, drug efficacy, or drug advertising.

The Drug Distributors

6. Products marketed by physician-owned repackaging companies should be considered unacceptable for reimbursement in any Medicare program except in those instances in which the

---

*In the original report this summary provided a page reference. That was not possible in this format.

Secretary of Health, Education, and Welfare determines that the availability of products marketed by such companies is in the public interest.

7. There is a need for medical associations, pharmacy associations, and consumer groups, working together at the local level, to develop mechanisms whereby patients may obtain information on local prescription prices, especially for long-term maintenance drugs.

The Drug Prescribers

8. Few practicing physicians seem inclined to voice any question of their competency in the field of therapeutic judgments. The ability of an individual physician to make sound judgments under quite confusing conditions, however, is now a matter of serious concern to leading clinicians, scientists, and medical educators.

Current American and Foreign Programs

9. In Medicaid and other State public assistance programs, no single method will by itself guarantee program efficiency, but without at least two features–reasonable formulary restrictions and effective data processing procedures–program controls will be ineffective. Although a co-payment requirement may not be widely acceptable in public assistance drug programs, its value in controlling costs in other programs seems evident.

10. Establishment of an out-of-hospital prescription drug program for the elderly or for other population groups has been shown to be economically feasible in many countries.

11. Rational prescribing, with due regard to quality of health care as well as to program costs, can be improved through the cooperation of physicians, pharmacists, drug manufacturers, and a governmental agency.

12. Reasonable program costs appear to be associated with (a) the use of a formulary developed by or in cooperation with the medical community, (b) the use of co-payment or co-insurance, (c) the use of utilization review procedures to prevent or minimize irrational prescribing, (d) the use of appropriate electronic or other data processing methods, with appropriate drug coding techniques, (e) simplified determination of beneficiary

eligibility, (f) population coverage which obviates the adverse selection of high-risk beneficiaries, (g) the use of a vendor payment formula based on actual acquisition cost verified by field audits rather than any catalog or wholesale list price, and (h) operation with the program serving as the legal purchasing agency, with utilization of competitive and negotiated bids, rather than merely as the reimbursing agency.

13. A permanent mechanism is needed at the Federal level to collect, analyze and exchange information, and to provide effective coordination of drug-related activities among the agencies involved.

Drug Quality

14. On the basis of available evidence, lack of clinical equivalency among chemical equivalents meeting all official standards has been grossly exaggerated as a major hazard to the public health.

15. The drug quality studies undertaken by the Food and Drug Administration are expected to be adequately if not completely up-to-date by 1971, and thus will provide reasonable assurance of uniform drug quality by that time.

16. There should be uniform standards of quality and efficacy for each drug in any federally-supported drug program. It would be inappropriate to provide for differential cost ranges for the products sold under brand or generic names.

Generic Prescribing and Drug Costs

17. The use of low-cost chemical equivalents can yield important savings, especially in the case of patients with cardiovascular disease, kidney disease, arthritis, and mental and nervous conditions. The use of such products should be encouraged wherever this is consistent with high-quality health care.

Formularies

18. In general, American physicians have found a formulary acceptable and practical, especially when it is designed by their clinical and scientific colleagues serving on expert committees, when quality is considered at least as important as price, when the formulary can be revised at appropriate intervals, and when there are provisions for prescribing unlisted drug products where special clinical conditions so demand.

19. The use of a formulary is not a mark of second-class medicine, but is, in fact, associated with the provision of the highest quality of medicine in the outstanding hospitals in the Nation.
20. Although use of a formulary is not a guarantee of high quality medical care, rational prescribing, effective utilization review, and control of costs, the achievement of these objectives in a drug program is difficult if not impossible without it.

Quality and Cost Standards

21. The exclusion of certain combination products, duplicative drugs, and noncritical products from Federal reimbursement would contribute significantly to rational prescribing, and moreover, it seems reasonable to assume this could yield overall savings of at least 10 percent.
22. Establishing product cost ranges reflecting the cost of drugs generally available by their generic names would save approximately 5 percent at the retail level.
23. Although significant program savings could be achieved through the application of techniques designed to improve the efficiency of vendor operations, it is impossible at this time to estimate the extent of these savings.
24. Considerable time would be required to develop all the necessary administrative mechanisms. Therefore full implementation of such provisions as applied to Federal reimbursement for prescribed drugs cannot be assured in less than two years after enactment of appropriate legislation.
25. Any necessary increases in Federal expenditures for the improvement of drug standards and quality control will have benefits which apply to all users of prescription drugs and should not be attached to the implementation of cost standards for drugs supplied in Federally-assisted programs.
26. Establishment of reasonable cost and charge ranges for drugs provided under the Medicare, Medicaid, and Maternal and Child Health programs is feasible, and would reduce the cost of drugs to the Federal and State governments without sacrifice of quality.

Drug Classification and Coding

27. Within a few years, it may be expected that prescription drug
    benefits under existing public and private programs will involve
    several hundred million prescriptions annually. Without a
    universal coding, classification and identification system–a
    common language for communicating essential information–
    the administrative and accounting costs for processing such a
    volume will inflate program costs beyond acceptable limits.

Utilization Review

28. There is an urgent need for further research to develop and test
    various approaches to effective utilization review–approaches
    which would be most acceptable to physicians, pharmacists,
    consumers and others, and which would obtain their effective
    support.

Drugs Under Medicare: The Issue
of Comprehensive Coverage

29. Because of the numerous and complex administrative problems
    and the high program costs involved in providing drug coverage
    under Medicare, it would be desirable–at least at the outset–to
    provide the benefit on a less-than-comprehensive basis.

Drugs Under Medicare: Coverage Under Part A
or Part B

30. While it would be feasible to provide coverage of out-of-hospital
    prescription drugs under either the hospital insurance (Part A) or
    medical insurance (Part B) programs of Medicare, there would
    be significant advantage, in terms of beneficiary eligibility and
    financing, in providing such coverage under the hospital
    insurance program.

Drugs Under Medicare: Alternative Proposals for Coverage

31. In order to achieve maximum benefits with whatever funds may
    be available, and to give maximum help to those of the elderly
    whose drug needs are the most burdensome, particular
    consideration should be given to providing coverage at the

outset mainly for those prescription drugs which are most likely to be essential in the treatment of serious long-term illness.

32. The use of an annual deductible to control costs presents opportunities that warrant further consideration.

33. Restricting benefits to those aged 70, 72, or more would reduce the size and cost of the program, but this is not a preferred approach at this time.

Drugs Under Medicare: Program Administration

34. It would be preferable for the vendor rather than the beneficiary to have major responsibility for keeping needed records and initiating claims, and to be reimbursed by the program.

35. Because of the large number of claims which would be involved, a suitable automated data processing system could play a vital role in claims processing and other administrative activities, and should be developed and adequately tested.

36. To the extent that appropriate utilization review methods are developed, these should be applied in a Medicare drug program.

Drugs Under Medicare: Program Reimbursement

37. Reimbursement for product cost, as one element in the total cost of a prescription, may be considered on the basis of (a) "usual and customary" charges, (b) listed wholesale price, (c) actual acquisition cost as verified by audit, or (d) a fixed program payment. Preference would be determined by the nature of the program.

38. Reimbursement for product cost should be based on the cost of the least expensive chemical equivalent of acceptable quality generally available on the market.

39. Since the expressed purpose of the social security program is to provide assistance to beneficiaries, wherever possible, within the framework of the existing health care system, the direct purchase of drugs by the Federal Government for Medicare beneficiaries is not recommended at this time, but this approach deserves further study.

40. The preferred method of reimbursing dispensing costs would depend on the nature of the program. If the program provides for a specific dispensing allowance to be paid to the drug vendor, rather than payment to the beneficiary, either a

percentage markup, or a fixed dispensing fee would be feasible, with a fixed fee approach being preferable.

41. Any drug insurance program instituted under Medicare should include cost-sharing provisions, such as co-payment or co-insurance.

42. Consideration should be given to the use of restrictions on maximum prescription quantities or on maximum prescription prices as additional cost-sharing approaches.

Organization of HEW Pharmaceutical Activities

43. No gain–and a substantial loss–in operating effectiveness would result from the organizational association of all pharmaceutical and related activities.

44. The drug development and screening programs of the National Institutes are integral parts of the biomedical research effort of the NIH and should remain the responsibility of these respective units.

45. The manpower development activities of the NIGMS (support of the pharmacology-toxicology centers) and of the Bureau of Health Manpower of the NIH are logical parts of the total responsibilities of these two units. Transfer of these activities to related activities of the FDA would not yield adequate benefits to warrant such an organizational change. The pharmaceutical-related activities of the Bureau of Manpower should be administered as part of the total effort to expand needed health manpower by that bureau.

46. The gathering, processing and dissemination of scientific information by the Consumer Protection and Environmental Health Service and its constituent, the Food and Drug Administration; by the National Library of Medicine; and by the National Institute of Mental Health are in each instance activities that flow logically out of other responsibilities of these units. These informational activities should be retained in their present organization.

47. The regulatory activities of the DBS are *not* logically a part of the biomedical research activities of the NIH. The DBS, however, does carry on research and drug development activities related to the central functions of the NIH, and it benefits materially from association with the research staffs of several Institutes of the NIH. Some advantages would be gained

by associating the regulatory activities of DBS with those of FDA. The DBS needs at times the regulatory skills of the FDA. But such transfer of the regulatory activities of DBS from NIH would result in the undesirable disassociation of these regulatory activities from the supporting research activities of NIH, and would cause a substantial loss in morale and probably a loss in key professional personnel. For these reasons, this action is not recommended.

48. No clearly apparent benefits could be derived from the separation of drug regulatory activities from food regulatory activities that would offset the economy and efficiency now achieved through the maintenance of closely related investigatory, research, and regulatory staffs.

SUMMARY OF RECOMMENDATIONS

The Drug Makers

1. The Department of Health, Education, and Welfare should conduct a continuing survey of drug costs, average prescription prices, and drug use.

2. The Secretary of Health, Education, and Welfare should call one or more conferences with representatives of the drug industry, pharmacy, clinical medicine, and consumer groups to consider–

   a. Provision of incentives to the drug industry to invest more research effort in products representing significant improvements to therapy and less in duplicative, noncontributory drug products and combinations.

   b. Development of a registration and licensing system under which no drug product would be permitted in interstate commerce unless produced under quality control standards set by the Secretary of Health, Education, and Welfare.

   c. Limitation of free drug samples, by industry agreement or legislation, to those specifically requested by prescribers.

   d. Development of more effective methods for ascertaining actual acquisition costs of prescription drugs.

3. The Secretary of Health, Education, and Welfare should call for a joint study by the Department of Health, Education, and

Welfare, the Department of Commerce, the Department of Justice, the Federal Trade Commission, and other Federal agencies to consider–

  a. The substantial differences in the prices at which drug products are offered to community pharmacies and to hospitals and government agencies.
  b. The substantial differences in the prices at which drug products are offered to American and foreign purchasers.
  c. Revision of current patent and trademark laws on prescription drugs.

The Drug Distributors

4. The Congress should enact legislation requiring that the containers of all dispensed prescription drugs be labeled with the identity, strength and quantity of the product, except where this is waived upon specific orders of the prescriber.
5. Encouragement should be given to the wider use of prepackage dispensing, in which manufacturers prepare and pharmacists dispense tablets and capsules in precounted form, in sealed, prelabeled containers, and in such numbers as conform to those most frequently prescribed by physicians.
6. The National Center for Health Services Research and Development should develop and support research to improve the efficiency and effectiveness of community and hospital pharmacy operations.
7. The Bureau of Health Manpower should support–

  a. The development of a pharmacist aide curriculum in junior colleges and other educational institutions.
  b. The development of appropriate curricula in medical and pharmacy schools for training pharmacists to serve as drug information specialists on the health team.
  c. A broad study of present and future requirements in pharmacy, adequacy of current pharmacy education, and the educational changes which must be made.

8. The Health Services and Mental Health Administration should support studies of state laws, regulations, and codes, with priority given to the establishment of model State licensing laws, uniform reciprocity standards, and provisions for the utilization of pharmacy aides.

The Drug Prescribers

9. The Department of Health, Education, and Welfare should provide expanded support to medical schools, enabling them to include a course in clinical pharmacology as an integral part of the medical curriculum.

10. The Department of Health, Education, and Welfare should establish or support a publication providing objective, up-to-date information and guidelines on drug therapy, based on the expert advice of the medical community.

11. The Department of Health, Education, and Welfare should support the efforts of county medical societies, pharmacy and therapeutics committees, medical foundations, and medical schools in taking the responsibility for providing continuing education to physicians on rational prescribing.

12. The Secretary of Health, Education, and Welfare should be authorized to publish and distribute a drug compendium listing all lawfully available prescription drugs, including such information as available dosage forms, clinical effects, indications and contraindications for use, and methods of administration, together with price information on each listed product, in readily accessible and comprehensive form.

Current American and Foreign Programs

13. The Federal Interdepartmental Health Policy Council should concern itself with the coordination of all ongoing Federal prescription drug purchase and reimbursement programs. A special subcommittee of the Council should be appointed for this purpose.

Drug Quality

14. The present clinical trials to determine the biological equivalency of important chemical equivalents should be continued by the Department of Health, Education, and Welfare on a high priority basis.

15. Adequate financial support should be provided to the Food and Drug Administration for necessary educational and inspection operations so that acceptable quality control methods can be instituted and properly maintained in all drug manufacturing and packaging establishments.

16. The Food and Drug Administration should be authorized to provide additional support, including grants-in-aid, to State and local agencies in order to improve quality control of prescription drugs in intrastate commerce.

Classification and Coding

17. The Department of Health, Education, and Welfare, the Department of Defense, and the Veterans Administration should test the proposed drug classification system to determine the feasibility of its eventual use in all public and private drug programs.
18. a. An appropriate identifying code number should be made part of all drug labels, package inserts, catalogs and advertising.
    b. An appropriate coding system should be developed and tested by government and industry for this purpose.
    c. After consideration of the results of this test, appropriate legislation should be introduced to require coding of all drug products in interstate commerce.
19. The drug code adopted by government and industry should be utilized in the National Drug Code Directory.

Utilization Review

20. The National Center for Health Services Research and Development, in cooperation with State and local medical groups, community pharmacies, hospitals, and consumer groups, should support pilot research projects on prescription drug utilization review methods.

Organization of HEW Pharmaceutical Activities

21. The present complex of activities now assigned to the Food and Drug Administration should continue to be administered by that agency.
22. The Social Security Administration should undertake continuing responsibility for the surveillance of drug costs, average prescription prices, and drug use.
23. Efforts should be strengthened to assure that the skills of experts both within and outside of the Department of Health,

Education, and Welfare are used to augment the scientific capabilities of the Food and Drug Administration.

24. Legislation should be enacted to authorize establishment within the Food and Drug Administration of a clinical and laboratory facility to provide the necessary opportunities for research by highly qualified basic scientists and clinicians.

25. The Secretary of Health, Education, and Welfare should, after consultation with representatives of the drug industry, pharmacy, clinical medicine, and consumer groups, appoint a study group to reappraise the efficiency of methods now used by the Division of Biologics Standards and the Food and Drug Administration to evaluate the safety and effectiveness of pharmaceuticals. The participants should direct attention to the appropriateness of the three existing classifications of pharmaceuticals–new drugs and "not new" drugs, certifiable products, and biologics. The study group should also consider the feasibility of developing a registration and licensing system which would assure that all drugs marketed in interstate commerce are produced under adequate quality control standards.

INTRODUCTION

On January 23, 1967, in his Older Americans Message to the Congress, President Lyndon B. Johnson focused national attention on the heavy burdens borne by many elderly men and women in attempting to pay the costs of prescription drugs. At the same time, he directed the Secretary of Health, Education, and Welfare to "undertake immediately a comprehensive study of the problems of including the cost of prescription drugs under Medicare."

Within this Department, informal studies in this complex and important area had already been underway for many months. These were quickly intensified by the President's directive.

On May 31, 1967, John W. Gardner–then Secretary of Health, Education, and Welfare–established the Task Force on Prescription Drugs. It consisted originally of four Assistant Secretaries, the Commissioner of Social Security, the Commissioner of Food and Drugs, the Acting Commissioner of Welfare, and the Surgeon General of the Public Health Service, with a specially-selected technical staff.

"The Task Force," he emphasized, "has no prior commitment to recommend for or against the inclusion of prescription drugs in the Medicare program. Its directive is first to investigate and then to make whatever recommendations it considers appropriate.

"The Task Force will examine a wide range of factors which are involved in the use of prescription drugs and will offer its recommendations within six months. The problems are numerous and complex. Some answers may be found speedily; others may take many months, possibly even years, of work, including laboratory research and clinical trials.

"In all of its work, I have asked the Task Force to measure the value of possible solutions not only in terms of dollars to be saved, but in the quality of health care to be delivered."

The scope and complexity of the assignment was by no means exaggerated by the Secretary. Inevitably, as formal operations were begun by the Task Force, and as additional information was requested by the Congress, it became essential to broaden the study to cover a large number of closely interrelated factors–the use of prescription drugs by the elderly, and their ability to meet drug expenses; the health needs of the elderly; the prescribing patterns of physicians, and the sources of drug information available to them; the nature of drug manufacture, and of drug promotion, drug advertising, drug pricing, and drug profits; the nature of drug distribution; the pharmacological aspects (including the hotly controversial matter of clinical equivalency); the role of formularies; the nature of current drug insurance programs, private and governmental, in this country and abroad; and the various alternatives involved in program financing, administration, reimbursement, classification, coding, and other aspects of drug insurance.

To undertake its studies in these and other fields, the Task Force enlisted the advice and guidance of many highly qualified experts, both governmental and nongovernmental. (A list of the non-governmental experts is presented at the end of this report.) We are most grateful to all of them for their invaluable assistance. None of them, of course, may be held responsible for any conclusions reached by the Task Force.

Because of the scope of these operations, no attempt was made to present final recommendations at the end of six months, as was originally contemplated. Instead, a series of five interim reports were published, beginning in March of 1968.

This Final Report contains most of the material published in interim form–much of it updated and expanded–together with some additional material.

It includes those findings which the Task Force believes to be particularly significant.

It includes recommendations for action–recommendations which, in some instances, are already being implemented by the various agencies of the Department.

Perhaps most significant are these:

- The finding that a drug insurance program under Medicare is needed by the elderly, and would be economically and medically feasible.
- The finding that the once-confusing matter of clinical equivalency is far less complex than had been anticipated, and that as a result of current laboratory and clinical studies–initiated in large part in response to requests by the Task Force–the problem is well on its way to solution.

In addition, much basic material–a substantial portion of it hitherto unavailable–has been obtained on various aspects of drug production, drug distribution, drug prescription, drug use, and drug insurance. This information appears to have great value for the Congress, many State and Federal governmental agencies, the medical and pharmacy communities, the drug industry, health insurance organizations, health educators, and consumer groups. It is being presented in a series of Task Force background papers, four of which have already been published and a fifth which is now in press.

It is our hope that all these publications–this Final Report and the background papers–will serve as the basis for careful analysis and discussion in the months and years to come.

More important, it is our hope that these publications, and the dedicated efforts of the many individuals who made them possible, will help to improve the health care not only for the elderly but for all Americans.

(Signed) Philip R. Lee, M.D.

CHAPTER 1
THE DRUG USERS

The elderly in the United States–those aged 65 or more–represent only a relatively small proportion–about 10 percent–of the total population of this country.

But their inordinate health needs, their high health care costs in general and high drug costs in particular, and their limited financial resources combine to create a serious and sometimes a devastating medical and economic problem far out of proportion to their numbers.

For many elderly people, illness serves as a major cause of their poverty by reducing their incomes, while poverty serves as a major contributory cause of illness by making it difficult for them to obtain adequate health care.

Yet it is not only the totally impoverished or the totally incapacitated who are in a precarious position. There are many elderly men and women who have some income and some savings–who may even have sufficient Medicare or other insurance to protect them against the bulk of hospital and medical costs of a brief illness–but who cannot pay for the out-of-hospital drugs and other costs of a long-continuing chronic illness without seeing their financial assets eroded or totally dissipated.

Numbers and Health Needs of the Elderly

There are now more than 19 million Americans over the age of 65. Among them, about 57 percent are women and 43 percent are men. This disproportion in sex distribution has been increasing steadily since about 1930–a trend of importance for any prescription drug study, since the use of these drugs by women is significantly higher than that by men.

In connection with the elderly, the term *aging* has often been considered synonymous with *illness*. There is, in fact, no necessary relationship between the two, but it is undeniably a fact that illness strikes the elderly far more frequently than it does younger age groups.

Approximately 80 percent of the elderly–in comparison with 40 percent of those under 65–suffer from one or more chronic diseases and conditions. Arthritis and rheumatism afflict 33 percent; heart disease, 17 percent; high blood pressure, 16 percent; other cardio-vascular ailments, 7.5 percent; mental and nervous conditions,

10.5 percent; hearing impairments, 22 percent; and visual problems, 15 percent.

Many of these conditions can be controlled or alleviated by modern medical care, especially by the proper use of drugs. This is reflected in the heavy expenses of the elderly for health care, and particularly in their heavy expenses for drugs.

Health Expenditures

Between 1950 and 1966, total national expenditures for health services and supplies–including hospital costs, physicians' fees, and drug costs–rose from $11.9 billion to $41.8 billion. (Per capita expenditures increased from $78.20 to $212.47.) In that same period, expenditures for out-of-hospital prescription drugs rose from $1.0 billion to $3.2 billion. (Per capita expenditures increased from $6.85 to $16.05.)

The increase in drug expenditures has resulted in part from a greater number of prescriptions per individual–an average of about 2.4 acquisitions per capita in 1950 and 4.6 in 1966–as well as from a significant rise in the average cost of prescriptions.

In 1950, a number of independent surveys reported the average cost of all prescriptions at the retail level was between $1.66 and $2.03. In 1966, independent surveys estimated the average was between $3.26 and $3.59. A special study conducted for the Task Force showed that the average prescription cost for the elderly in 1966 was even higher–$3.91.

Distribution of Drug Expenditures

If drug use were equally distributed among all groups–that is, 4 to 5 prescriptions per year at a cost of $3 to $4–there would be no major problem for the elderly. But this is far from the actual situation.

Although the elderly represent slightly less than 10 percent of the total population, they account for about 22 percent of all out-of-hospital prescriptions and about 25 percent of all out-of-hospital prescription drug expenditures.

A nationwide study by the National Center for Health Statistics in fiscal year 1965 showed the following (see Table 1):

- The average number of acquisitions–i.e., the number of prescriptions or refills–for the elderly was more than twice that for the total population, and nearly three times that for those under 65.

- The average number of acquisitions for elderly women was nearly 50 percent more than the number for men.
- The per capita expenditure for prescription drugs for the elderly was almost three times greater than that for the total population, and more than three times greater than that for those under 65.
- The per capita expenditure for elderly women was more than one-third higher than that for elderly men.
- The per capita expenditure for the elderly with severe disabilities was nearly three times greater than that for those with no disabilities.

These 1964-65 data indicate that for the relatively few elderly with no chronic conditions, the annual cost for prescribed medicines was $3.60 per capita. For those with one or more chronic conditions, the number of acquisitions rose to 13.5 and the annual cost to $48.80.

TABLE 1. Average Number of Acquisitions and Annual Cost of Prescribed Drugs, Per Person by Selected Characteristics, Fiscal Year 1965.

Characteristics	No. of Acquisitions[a]			Annual Cost		
	All Ages	Under 65	65 and Over	All Ages	Under 65	65 and Over
All Persons	4.7	4.0	11.4	$15.40	$12.77	$41.40
Sex						
Male	3.7	3.1	9.3	12.00	9.88	34.70
Female	5.6	4.8	13.1	18.60	15.49	46.70
Color						
White	4.9	4.2	11.5	16.40	13.62	42.60
Nonwhite	3.1	2.7	10.2	7.80	6.57	26.90
Geographic Region						
Northeast	4.4	3.8	10.6	13.30	10.80	37.00
North Central	4.4	3.8	10.9	15.00	12.37	39.90
South	5.3	4.5	13.6	17.50	14.64	47.40
West	4.3	3.7	9.7	15.30	12.93	40.00
Disability–Men						
None				14.80		19.40
Mild				33.50		40.90
Moderate				33.60		40.80
Severe				71.70		71.00
Disability–Women						
None				23.20		34.00
Mild				50.00		64.40
Moderate				63.40		67.60
Severe				101.40		94.70

[a] New prescriptions or refills.

When the condition was sufficiently severe to limit major activity completely, acquisitions averaged 21.7 prescriptions, and costs averaged $78.80. Similarly, the average cost of a prescription was higher for persons with chronic conditions–$3.60 for persons with no such conditions, $4 for those with one or more conditions, and $4.10 for those with complete limitation in their major activity. The data also indicated that prescription expenses of those of the elderly with severe chronic conditions–about 15 percent of all elderly persons–were over 6 times as great as the expenses of younger people.

In general, the survey showed, total prescription drug expenditures in all age groups were higher for women than for men, for whites than for nonwhites, and for those in the South and West. The higher expenditures for whites appear to be a reflection of their greater affluence–their greater ability to seek medical care and to afford drugs rather than greater health needs. The high costs in the South appear to be related to exceptionally heavy utilization, while in the West they reflect lower utilization but much higher costs per prescription.

Similarly, although the burden of drug costs falls most heavily upon the elderly, it does not fall evenly upon these individuals.

A 1968 estimate, for example, indicates that 20 percent of the elderly will have no drug expenses, while the costs will be less than $50 for 41.5 percent, between $50 and $99 for 19 percent, between $100 and $249 for 15.5 percent, and $250 or more for 4 percent.

A recent investigation, carried out on a limited group in Pennsylvania, indicated that, among the elderly who actually obtained prescription drugs, about 2 percent accounted for about 21 percent of the total cost, and about 10 percent of the individuals accounted for about 47 percent of the cost.

An earlier study by the National Health Survey in 1962 of the expenses for prescription and nonprescription drugs found that 24 percent of the elderly had no drug expenses, 40 percent had annual expenses which were less than $50, 17 percent had expenses between $50 and $99, and 18 percent had expenses of $100 or more. Among these 18 percent, the expenses were $100 to $249 for 14.7 percent, $250 to $499 for 2.9 percent, and $500 or more for 0.5 percent.

Financial Resources of the Elderly

The size of drug bills for the elderly represents only one phase of the problem. Intimately related is their ability to pay those bills.

Since July 1, 1966, implementation of the Medicare program has substantially increased the ability of many elderly men and women to meet their doctor and hospital bills, not entirely but in large part. Expenditures for out-of-hospital prescription drugs, however, are not covered by the present Medicare law, and it has been necessary for elderly patients to utilize other sources.

Income. In 1966, half of the families headed by an elderly individual had total incomes–including Social Security payments–of less than $3,645, or $70 a week. For elderly men and women living alone, or with someone not a relative, more than half had incomes of less than $1,500, or about $30 a week.

In spite of recent improvements in OASDI benefit levels, the elderly remain among the most impoverished groups in the population. It is estimated that as of January 1, 1969, almost 3 million elderly persons were living in poor households, as measured by the Social Security Administration's poverty index. Counting also elderly persons in institutions and those with incomes below the poverty level who are living in households whose total income is above that level, a little over 7 million elderly persons, or 36 percent of the total elderly population, were poor.

Among social security beneficiaries, although benefit income kept some 6.8 million out of poverty, another 5.8 million or 36 percent remained poor. An additional 3 million were in the near-poor group, only a little better off.

Assets. Recent studies have shown that the average per capita amount of savings and other assets held by the elderly is about $15,000.

But 30 percent of the elderly have assets of less than $1,000 apiece. For them, a serious illness could wipe out their meager savings in a few months.

Health Insurance. Health insurance through Blue Cross, Blue Shield, commercial insurance companies, group practice plans and other organizations is available to many of those over the age of 65, but provision of prescription drugs–except to hospitalized patients–is limited.

Where out-of-pocket drug expenses are covered, these are generally included in major medical policies involving deductibles of $100, $250, or $500–useful only in so-called "catastrophic" illnesses.

Recently, drug insurance programs have been developed to provide adequate coverage of out-of-hospital drug costs, but membership in the plans is usually limited to members of employed groups, and few of these are in the older-age group.

As of the end of 1966, while about 51 percent of the elderly had some form of hospital insurance complementary to Medicare, only about 9 percent had insurance coverage for their out-of-hospital prescription drugs; drug coverage ranked below private-duty nursing, visiting-nurse services and nursing-home care in extent of coverage.

Tax Relief. To the extent that expenses for drugs are included as deductions on income tax returns, reduced income tax payments represent a source of payment for these drugs.

For the elderly, such relief obtained through Federal income tax deductions has been estimated to represent about 8 percent of drug expenditures. But these savings benefit only those elderly individuals who receive enough income to require income tax payments, and would be of little importance to those with low incomes. Data are not available on the extent of such savings achieved through deductions on State income taxes.

Free Drugs. From the 1964-65 study of the National Center for Health Statistics, it appears that about 3 percent of the elderly received their drugs at no cost from their physicians.

Public Assistance. About 6 percent in 1964-65 obtained prescription drugs from State or local welfare agencies or similar sources. The provision of free drugs through welfare agencies–under Medicaid or other Federal, State or local programs–may solve the problem as it directly affects some of the elderly. The basic economic problem is not solved, however, but merely shifted from the elderly to the taxpayers.

It is estimated that in calendar year 1967, the latest year for which figures are available, expenditures for drugs for elderly persons through State vendor payment drug programs for welfare recipients in the Federally-aided public assistance categories totalled about $105 million. The Federal share of these payments was about 53 percent. About 1.3 million older people received these benefits, which are payable under 41 State or territorial assistance programs. In addition, several of the assistance programs included an allowance for drug costs in their cash payments to older people.

Out-of-Pocket Costs. In enabling the elderly to meet their out-of-hospital prescription drug expenses, the combined impact of insurance coverage, tax relief, free drugs, and public assistance does not seem to be substantial, covering only about 20 percent of total costs.

The remainder–about 80 percent–must be met by out-of-pocket expenditures from income and assets. For those over 65, these financial resources are rarely substantial.

Thus, the elderly, with limited income, limited savings, and minimal protection from health insurance and other sources, are obliged to face the burdens of drug costs which are far heavier on a per capita basis than those which weigh on their fellow citizens, who in most cases are not only younger, but also healthier and wealthier.

Patterns of Drug Use by the Elderly

Essential for an effective attack against the drug problems of the elderly are detailed, objective data on the drugs they actually use and the costs of these prescriptions.

In 1966, for example, the elderly obtained about 225 million out-of-hospital prescriptions at a total retail cost of almost $900 million, involving many thousands of different drug products. But this knowledge is not enough.

It is necessary to know–

- which drugs, by brand or generic name, were dispensed for the elderly;
- which were utilized most frequently;
- which diseases accounted for the greatest drug utilization;
- which drugs were most frequently involved in long-term maintenance therapy;
- how much each of these drugs cost at the wholesale level, and at the retail level; and
- to what extent drug costs could be reduced if low-cost chemical equivalents were used wherever they were available.

To obtain the needed information, the Task Force requested the Public Health Service to undertake a special study, with major responsibility assigned to the Health Economics Branch of the Division of Medical Care Administration, and assistance provided by other agencies within the Bureau of Health Services, and by the Food and Drug Administration.

The project–probably the first of its kind ever undertaken–was aimed at developing a master list of the drugs which were most frequently prescribed and dispensed for the elderly in 1966, and which would account for about four-fifths of their drug use during that year.

The Task Force Master Drug List. As developed for the Task Force, the Master Drug List (MDL) contained the 409 most frequently prescribed drugs dispensed to the elderly in 1966. These accounted for 174.7 million, or 88 percent, of all prescriptions dispensed by community pharmacies for the elderly in that year, and for $682.3 million, or 88 percent, of their prescription drug costs at the retail level.

Included among the 409 products were 379 which were dispensed under their brand names. These accounted for more than 90 percent of the total number of MDL prescriptions, about 90 percent of the total acquisition cost to retailers, and 95 percent of the total retail cost to patients.

Among these were 86 products which were dispensed under their brand names, but for which chemical equivalents were available–often but not always at lower cost–and could have been prescribed under generic names. They accounted for about 29 percent of the total number of prescriptions, 27 percent of the total acquisition cost to retailers, and 27 percent of the retail cost to patients.

Also included were 30 drugs which were dispensed under their generic names. They accounted for about 10 percent of the number of prescriptions, 10 percent of the total acquisition cost, and 5 percent of the total retail cost.

Average Prescription Cost. For all 409 MDL drugs, the average cost per prescription was $3.91. For the 379 drugs dispensed under brand name, it was $4.11. For the 30 drugs dispensed under generic name, it was $2.02.

Most Widely Used Drugs. The 10 most frequently used products–headed by an oral antidiabetic agent, and including two tranquilizers, two diuretics, an analgesic, an anti-arthritic agent, a cardiac drug, and two sedatives–accounted for 20 percent of the total number of MDL prescriptions, 21.6 percent of the total acquisition cost to retailers, and 20.7 percent of the total retail price to consumers.

Only two of these were available from several manufacturers under a generic name.

Approximately 50 percent of the total cost to patients was represented by the top 53 drugs, which also represented 53 percent of the total number of prescriptions and 49 percent of the total acquisition cost to retailers. Among these were 30 drugs which could be obtained only under a brand name from a single supplier, 16 which were dispensed under a brand name although a chemical equivalent was available, and 7 which were dispensed under generic name.

Therapeutic Category. Cardiovascular preparations–including vasodilators, digitalis and its congeners, and hypotensive drugs– accounted for 38.9 million, or 22 percent, of the total prescriptions, and $157.8 million, or 23 percent, of the total retail cost to consumers.

Tranquilizers, with 16.9 million prescriptions at a total cost of $78.9 million, rated second, followed by diuretics, with 16.0 million prescriptions at $62.6 million; and sedatives, with 15.1 million prescriptions at $32.3 million.

These four categories together represented about one-half of all prescriptions for products in the MDL, and of the total cost to patients.

Antibiotics ranked fifth, including 13 million prescriptions at a retail cost of $64.3 million.

Diagnostic Category. About 66.2 million, or 38 percent, of the total prescriptions, at a cost of $244.3 million, or 36 percent, of the total retail cost, were used for the treatment of heart disease and hypertension.

An additional 17.3 million prescriptions, at a retail cost of $65.4 million, were applied for the control of arthritis and rheumatism.

About 11.6 million prescriptions, at a cost of $47.4 million, were dispensed for the treatment of mental and nervous conditions.

Together these groups accounted for 95.1 million, or 54 percent, of the total MDL prescriptions, and $357 million, or 52 percent, of the total cost to consumers.

Maintenance Therapy. A sizeable proportion of out-of-hospital drugs prescribed for the elderly are so-called long-term maintenance drugs, used primarily for the control of chronic diseases. Few of these–at least at the present state of knowledge–can be cured, but in many instances appropriate drug therapy will enable the patient to live a reasonably comfortable and productive life.

Among the 409 drugs in the MDL, 70 were prescribed for 30 to 59 days during the year, 42 of them for 60 to 89 days, and 78 of them for 90 days or more.

These last 78 accounted for only about 20 percent of all MDL products, but they represented 59.6 million, or 34 percent, of all MDL prescriptions, and $242 million, or 35 percent, of total costs to the consumer. More than half of them were for the control of cardiovascular disease.

From the foregoing, the Task Force finds that the requirements for appropriate prescription drug therapy by the elderly are very great–far greater, in fact, than those of any other group–and that many elderly men and women are now unable to meet these needs with their limited incomes, savings, or present insurance coverage. Their inability to afford the drugs they require may well be reflected in needless sickness and disability, unemployability, and costly hospitalization which could have been prevented by adequate out-of-hospital treatment.

With steadily increasing prescription expenditures, this problem is destined to become increasingly serious.

We recognize that Medicare provides the great majority of the elderly with substantial protection covering the drugs they receive while they are inpatients in hospitals and extended care facilities, and that they therefore have adequate protection against the drug expenses associated with their most serious acute illnesses, but they have a need for improved protection against the cost of drugs they use when they are not hospital or extended care inpatients, and especially against those costs associated with the serious chronic conditions which afflict them.

We therefore find that, in order to improve the access of the elderly to high quality health care, and to protect them where possible against high drug expenses which they may be unable to meet, there is need for an out-of-hospital drug insurance program under Medicare.

CHAPTER 2
THE DRUG MAKERS

Since World War II, the American drug industry has risen to a position of worldwide leadership in drug research, development, production, and distribution.

It is now the center of intense controversy, and heavy criticism has been leveled at both its motives and its methods. At the same time, it has been vigorously defended, with detailed descriptions of its many contributions to the health of mankind, and with insistence on the reasonableness of its prices and profits.

The Industry

Total drug sales–prescription and nonprescription drugs alike–have increased substantially in the last decade, rising from nearly $3 billion in 1957 to about $5 billion in 1967 at the manufacturer's level. Prescription drugs accounted for about two-thirds of this volume.

Foreign drug sales by American companies exceeded a billion dollars in 1967.

Approximately 95 percent of the prescription drug sales were made by the 136 member companies that comprise the Pharmaceutical Manufacturers Association (PMA). Members of the PMA produce and sell both brand-name and generic-name products. Just as they account for the overwhelming proportion of sales, they conduct essentially all of the industry's research, they control the overwhelming proportion of drug patents, they conduct the most vigorous promotion of their products, they compete vigorously–usually on the basis of innovation and quality and rarely on the basis of price–for the favor of the medical profession, and they achieve the industry's highest rates of profit.

The remaining five percent of the Nation's prescription drugs are manufactured by many hundreds of companies, and are sold under both brand and generic names. The total number of such firms is believed to be more than 700. They control few drug patents, do little or no research, compete on the market on the basis of both quality and price, conduct only minimal promotion of their products, and achieve relatively low rates of profit.

Research and Development

Various Federal agencies support drug-related research and development at the rate of more than $100 million a year. In addition, other studies included in the Federally-supported biomedical research program may be expected to have eventual implications for drug research and development.

The drug industry's research and development program is now nearly $500 million a year, almost all conducted by about 70 of the PMA members.

The industry's research effort has been noteworthy in many respects–

- New drugs developed through research have given physicians remarkable weapons for the improved treatment of infections, metabolic disorders, arthritis, heart disease, high blood pressure, and a host of other crippling or deadly diseases.

- Based on percentage of sales, the drug industry's investment in research is about three times greater than that of any other major industry.
- The number of new products has been impressive. For example, between 1957 and 1968, 311 products introduced on the market were described as important new single entities. They represented about 15 percent of the 2,131 new prescription drug products introduced during that period. Also included were 1,440 products containing two or more older drugs in a new combination, and 380 drugs which were essentially duplicates or minor modifications of products already in use.
- The annual number of important new entities, those which represent significant advances, reached a peak in 1959–three years before the Kefauver-Harris Drug Amendments of 1962–and decreased steadily until 1967, when the number started to rise again.

Also impressive is the vigor and frequency with which industry spokesmen have said that any government interference in their operations may force them to reduce their research programs.

The Task Force is convinced that the directions and quality of some industry research programs deserve careful consideration.

We have noted the serious and increasing concern expressed by practicing physicians, medical educators, pharmacologists, and economists–and even some industry leaders–at the number of molecular modifications of older drugs introduced each year. Some of these modifications undoubtedly represent significant advances, but most appear to be so called "me-too" drugs–substances which are not significantly different from other drugs, nor significantly better, and represent little or no improvement in therapy, but which are sufficiently manipulated in chemical structure to win a patent.

We have noted the comparable concern expressed at the number of new fixed combinations of old drugs introduced each year. Although these combinations may offer some convenience to elderly patients in particular, clinicians and pharmacologists have cautioned that they also involve obvious hazards and combine drugs in a "locked-in" proportion which may or may not fill the needs of individual patients.

The numbers of duplicative and combination drug products introduced in recent years have been decreasing, but they still represent the great majority of all so-called new drugs.

It is evident that these duplicative products, along with combination products, are used widely by some physicians, perhaps on the basis of the industry's exceedingly effective marketing and promotion activities. For example, of the 409 most frequently dispensed drugs for the elderly included in the Task Force Master Drug List, about 190 are combination products, and a substantial number of the others could be classed as duplicative or "me-too" products. But it is also evident that the need for this overabundance of drug products has not been convincing to some medical experts. Thus, in many of the Nation's leading hospitals, when expert physicians have served on pharmacy and therapeutics committees to select the drugs needed for both inpatient and outpatient therapy, they have generally found many if not most of these duplicative drugs and combinations to be unnecessary. These products have been found generally unnecessary by physicians providing medical care to the armed forces. They have been found generally unnecessary by leading clinical pharmacologists.

If these items were offered at prices substantially lower than the products they duplicate, they would provide at least an economic advantage, but in most instances they are introduced at the same or even higher prices.

The development of such duplicative drugs or combination products cannot be considered an inexpensive fringe benefit. Each requires laboratory research, clinical trials and the accumulation of sufficient data to demonstrate to the Food and Drug Administration that the new product–although it may not represent any significant therapeutic advance–is at least safe and efficacious.

Since important new chemical entities represent only a fraction–perhaps 10 to 25 percent–of all new products introduced each year, and the remainder consists merely of minor modifications or combination products, then the Task Force finds that much of the drug industry's research and development activities would appear to provide only minor contributions to medical progress.

We likewise find that to the extent the industry directs a share of its research program to duplicative, noncontributory products, there is a waste of skilled research manpower and research facilities, a waste of clinical facilities needed to test the products, a further confusing proliferation of drug products which are promoted to physicians, and a further burden on the patient or taxpayer who, in the long run, must pay the costs.

A solution to this problem requires joint efforts on the parts of industry and the Federal Government.

Quality Control

Any company, large or small, brand-name or generic-name producer, can institute and maintain an effective quality control program, and most companies have apparently done so. The cost of such a program has been estimated to be about 2.4 percent of sales for a large company, but may be somewhat more for a smaller firm.

On the other hand, not all companies have maintained adequate quality control, and their products have had to be recalled–either voluntarily or by government order–for such defects as mislabeling, subpotency, or contamination. These recalls have involved both large and small firms, and both brand-name and generic-name products.

Several hundred such violations are reported each year. Investigations have often indicated that these are related to the failure of a manufacturer to comply with what are known as Good Manufacturing Practices, including such factors as plant sanitation, personnel surveillance, equipment maintenance, raw material standards, record keeping, and quality checks at every appropriate stage of manufacture and packaging.

The Task Force believes that this situation may be substantially improved by the intensified inspection program introduced in 1968 by the Food and Drug Administration. At the same time, it believes that further study is warranted of the alternative proposal that a registration and licensing system be established under which no drug product would be permitted in interstate commerce unless produced under quality standards set by the Secretary of Health, Education, and Welfare.

Marketing

For those major companies which have presented any data, marketing expenses–including particularly those for advertising and promotion–represent from about 15 to 35 percent of sales. Such expenses for generic-name products appear to be substantially lower than those for brand-name products.

Industry spokesmen have claimed that marketing is an accepted part of any business activity; that their marketing costs are reasonable; and that their marketing efforts–including advertising, direct mailings, and personal visits by detail men to physicians–are primarily educational in nature. They have claimed that the promotional aspects of drug marketing are a mark of the intense competition in the industry.

On the other hand, critics have asserted that intensive promotional efforts may be acceptable to sell such products as detergents, beer and used automobiles, but not for such vital necessities as prescription drugs; that the expenses for drug marketing are excessive and add needlessly to the cost of prescriptions; that prescription drug advertising and other promotion has reached the proportions of supersaturation, and that some has been–at least until recent regulations were established by the Food and Drug Administration–inaccurate, unscientific and biased.

It appears evident to the Task Force that drug promotional activities are related to the particular type of competition which unquestionably exists in the prescription drug industry–among others, an intense competition between companies, with the promise of a greater share of a relatively limited market and richer profits for the successful competitor–but that these activities have little to do with normal price competition in the retail marketplace, with the promise of eventual price savings to the consumer.

The Strategy of Names. Intimately related to marketing, and the competition between brand and generic products, is the subject of brand and generic names.

In the past, whether fortuitously or by design, most generic names–though certainly not all of them–have been relatively long, complicated and difficult to pronounce and remember.

During the past year, this situation has improved somewhat as the result of new policies established by the U.S. Adopted Names Council, but more improvement is needed.

The Task Force commends the Council for its efforts toward simplifying generic names and urges that these efforts be continued and strengthened.

Advertising and Promotion. Included among the promotional activities of some major prescription drug companies have been the support of scientific or medical conferences or symposia totally unrelated to any commercial product; the publication of educational materials for the public on such subjects as prevention of narcotic and drug abuse, immunization campaigns, and school health; the establishment of scholarships and fellowships, especially for the benefit of underdeveloped countries; and the no-strings-attached support of some scientific and medical societies.

These and similar activities are held in high esteem by many in the scientific and medical community, and are viewed as significant contributions to the improvement of public health.

Also included among promotional activities is the drug advertising in medical journals, direct mailings, throw-away publications, and others which has long since reached astounding proportions. It is estimated that the major drug companies together spent in 1968 some $4,500 per physician annually to reach each of the nearly 200,000 physicians who represent the target audience–those who will decide for which drug product their patients should pay.

Significantly, this advertising rarely if ever mentions price.

Unquestionably, much of this material is accurate and educational. The frequency of biased, inaccurate drug advertising has apparently been reduced since the enforcement of new advertising regulations by the Food and Drug Administration began in 1967. But the overall value of such advertising volume continues to be seriously questioned.

Similarly, the potential impact of these large advertising expenditures on the editorial policies of the journals which are supported in large part by drug advertisements appears to deserve careful study.

Detail Men. Major brand-name manufacturers–and a few generic-name companies–employ about 20,000 representatives to call on physicians, hospital, and pharmacists, and provide information on their products.

Whether such activities may be described as primarily promotional or primarily educational is difficult to determine. It is doubtful, however, that physicians can expect such detail men to give invariably unprejudiced and objective advice.

Significantly, the presentations of detail men rarely include mention of price.

Free Samples. Free drug samples have customarily been distributed to physicians without request to induce them to try a product and test its advantages on their own patients. But few physicians are able to undertake any serious trials of this nature. Furthermore, if a physician does try a drug, in most instances he can do so with only a very few patients; the possibility that such a limited study can serve as a basis for a scientific judgment seems to be small.

Free drug samples have made it possible for physicians and

hospitals to supply drugs at no cost to some indigent patients. This need, however, has been modified by the advent of Medicaid and other programs under which Federal and State welfare funds may be used to provide drugs to eligible patients.

It has been reported that free samples have been involved in accidental poisonings, drug abuse, and black market activities.

Some major drug manufacturers have reacted to this problem by distributing free samples only to those prescribers who have specifically requested them. It appears that further steps in this direction call for joint efforts by the industry and the Federal Government.

Industry Prices

Few aspects of the drug industry are more confused–or more confusing–than its pricing structure. Ostensibly, wholesale prices are listed in company catalogs and price lists, but these generally represent maximum prices. They serve merely as an umbrella beneath which actual prices are set by quantity discounts, hospital discounts, government discounts, two-for-the-price-of-one deals, rebates, and other special arrangements.

With many Federal, State and private drug programs now using reimbursement formulas supposedly based on product costs to the vendor, there is need for developing an efficient system to ascertain actual acquisition costs. This calls for cooperation among manufacturers, wholesalers, vendors, insurance companies, and governmental agencies.

Price Indices. Particular confusion has resulted from the comparison of various indices intended to indicate the trend of drug costs.

From the Consumer Price Index of the Bureau of Labor Statistics, it seems obvious that retail drug prices have been decreasing steadily since about 1958.

From three independent surveys, it seems equally obvious that these prices have been increasing during the same period.

The disparity is based on the fact that the indices are measuring different things.

The BLS index is aimed at measuring the change in a relatively fixed "market basket" of about a dozen arbitrarily selected drug products. During the past decade, the prices of these items have, on the average, decreased. The items selected for the "basket," however, do not accurately and fully represent the most widely used drugs, and they do not reflect the changes in consumer expenditures which constantly occur when new, presumably better, and certainly more costly products are introduced on the market and replace less costly products.

On the other hand, the independent, surveys are not concerned with the price changes of any individual drug products, but instead are aimed at determining the average price of all the prescriptions which people do purchase. All three of these surveys show a definite upward trend in the average cost of these prescriptions, but they do not agree in the extent of increase because of different sampling methods.

Thus, there is need for information on actual drug costs, expenses and utilization by the elderly and other groups.

Accordingly, we recommend that the Department of Health, Education, and Welfare should conduct a continuing survey of drug costs, average prescription prices, and drug use.

Hospital and Government Discounts. Many drug manufacturers customarily offer their products to hospitals at prices substantially lower than those available to community pharmacists. The savings are not necessarily reflected in lower drug prices to hospital patients.

To a considerable extent, these hospital discounts represent a subsidy to hospital patients–or, more often, to the hospitals themselves–at the expense of nonhospitalized patients.

Spokesmen for some pharmacy associations have urged that wholesale prices to hospital pharmacies and community pharmacies be kept at the same level–a move which would lower prices moderately to community pharmacies, but raise them substantially to hospital pharmacies. Hospital spokesmen have declared any such action would raise hospital per diem rates still higher.

Similar differences are apparent between the prices of drugs sold to community pharmacies and those sold to Federal and State agencies.

The Task Force believes that the substantial differences in the prices at which the same drug products are offered to community pharmacies and to hospitals and governmental agencies, respectively, deserve further examination.

Foreign Prices. Many American companies offer their products for sale in foreign countries at prices substantially below those available in the United States primarily to meet price competition which does not generally exist in this country.

During the past few years, there has been mounting insistence that these companies should price their products essentially the same in all countries.

The drug companies have countered that any increase in their foreign prices would drive them out of the foreign markets, not only reducing their earnings but upsetting still further this country's unfavorable balance of trade. On the other hand, any attempt to reduce American prices to the level of prices on foreign markets could be catastrophic to their total financial structure.

We believe that further study is required on the different prices at which drug products are offered to American and foreign purchasers.

Patents, Trademarks and Competition

In the case of most commodities, rival companies compete vigorously on the open market on the basis of both quality and price, with the consumer having the right to make the final judgment. In most instances, the results have been steadily increasing quality and decreasing price.

In the case of drugs, there are distinct differences. The competition is based almost entirely on real or presumed therapeutic advantages. The patient, who must pay for the drug, rarely has any voice in its selection. The decision on which product the patient must buy is made by the physician. Although moderate or even enormous price differences may exist between products of comparable quality, this is seldom brought to the physician's attention.

Some have attempted to justify this situation by describing the physician as the patient's expert purchasing agent. In the view of the Task Force, this concept is not valid; in most situations, a purchasing agent who purchased without consideration of both quality and price would be unworthy of trust.

In what has been described as this "new competition" in the drug business, patents and trademarks have played key roles.

On the one hand, industry supporters have insisted that the present patent and trademark system makes possible the incentives and rewards that are essential for the industry's large research and development effort, the flow of new products to which it leads, the subsequent benefit to health, and the ready identification of brand-name products.

On the other, it has been asserted that drug patents, combined with multi-million-dollar drug advertising campaigns, can keep new or small companies out of the high-profit circle, and effectively stifle price competition in the marketplace.

Various proposals to modify the patent system have been considered by the Task Force.

Abolition of Drug Patents. Removal of all patent protection from new drugs, it appears, would be a destructive move. Virtually all the important new drugs of recent years have come from countries providing patent protection. Few, if any, have come from Eastern European nations which offer little or no patent protection. Several important drugs have originated in Italy, which does not provide patent protection, but these have been quickly patented in foreign countries.

Restricted Patent Life. It has been estimated that a company will usually recoup all its research and development costs of a product within about three years after it reaches the market. Accordingly, it has been proposed that the patent on a drug should be reduced from the present period of 17 years to a much briefer period–such as 10 years, 7 years, or even 5 years.

It has been shown, however, that requirements to establish the safety and efficacy of a new drug may take many years of effort–perhaps as many as seven years. Where such testing continues after a patent is issued, the period of actual patent protection may be less than the statutory 17-year period.

Co-Terminal Patents and Trademarks. It has also been recommended that the patent life on a drug be maintained at the present 17 years, but that exclusive rights to the trademark should last no longer than the patent. Thus, at the end of the 17-year period, any qualified manufacturer would be free to market the drug under its original trademark or brand name.

Generic Name Only. A related proposal is that new drugs should be marketed only under a generic name–exclusively by the inventor until the patent expired, and then by any qualified manufacturer who desired to produce it. Used with the generic name would be the name of the manufacturer, to identify the source of the product. This would clearly tend to minimize the confusing multiplicity and complexity of names put before physicians and would better identify the nature of the drug.

Compulsory Licensing. Unlike the United States, many countries have provisions under which the government may require the patent holder to license other manufacturers through a suitable royalty system. These provisions have rarely been enforced, perhaps because realistic price competition exists in the marketplace and lower prices may be invoked through negotiations.

Proponents of such legislation in this country have argued that if licensing were required after the first three years of a product's market life–i.e., after major recovery of research and development costs–other firms could enter that product market by paying royalties, and price competition might then occur among these rivals. Beneficial results to consumers would be possible only for those products with a commercial life longer than three years. For such products, the patent holder would continue to earn an innovator's profits, though perhaps at lower rates than before, and consumers possibly could purchase prescriptions at lower price levels.

Make-or-Sell Licensing. As yet another approach, it has been proposed that the patent holder should not be permitted to monopolize both the manufacture, and the sale of a new drug, but should be required to license either other producers or other sellers.

We note that these and other proposals to amend patent and trademark laws on drugs have been considered in the United States and other countries, and believe further study is necessary.

Release of Technical Information

As part of the New Drug Application procedure of the Food and Drug Administration, the manufacturer of a new drug product is required to submit a voluminous quantity of clinical and technical information, including data on ingredients and methods of production.

The FDA had held that the New Drug Application and the technical information included in it are the property of the applicant, and cannot be released–except with the applicant's consent–even after the patent has expired.

Whether or not this policy is appropriate and in the public interest has been questioned. Recently Dr. James L. Goddard, then Commissioner of the Food and Drug Administration, testified on this matter:

> ". . . I think properly that the question should be discussed by Congress in terms of the scientific and business community involved. Congress should get down to the issues involved here and see whether or not the interest of the public at large might better be served by a public policy which permitted disclosure of the clinical [and] the scientific information incorporated in New Drug Applications."

Profits and Risks

In a free enterprise system, it is obvious that a company must make a profit. Unless it achieves this primary objective, it cannot stay in business.

Ample evidence is available to demonstrate that the drug industry has been able to stay in business. It has maintained an annual profit rate based on net worth which is substantially above that of the average of major American industries.

- One study of 41 industries has shown that, between 1956 and 1966, the drug industry never ranked lower than third on the basis of after-tax income as a percentage of net worth. In six of those years, it ranked in first place.
- Another study showed that, among 31 major industries, drug makers have averaged an 18.1 percent return on capital, as compared with 9.7 percent for the whole group.

A similar high rate of profit for the drug industry is indicated on the basis of profits calculated as a percentage of sales.

Spokesmen for the drug industry have agreed that its profitability is above average. They say, however, that this high rate is necessitated by the high degree of risk in the industry, and the need to attract the capital to finance further growth.

The Task Force has been unable to find sufficient evidence to support the concept of the drug industry as a particularly risky enterprise.

There is abundant evidence that the development of an individual drug may be associated with a high degree of risk, and that any such development is an economic as well as a scientific gamble.

There is, however, no evidence that this kind of risk characterizes a typical major drug company with a substantial line of drug products. When such a company undergoes a painful loss in this kind of a gamble, the record would seem to show, it generally covers it by substantial profits on other drugs.

The record would also tend to show that–at least during the past 20 years–losses of this nature have driven few if any major pharmaceutical manufacturers into serious financial straits.

In recent years, some major American drug manufacturers have diversified their operations by moving into other operations. In some instances, this has been described as an attempt to minimize risks. At the same time, however, it is apparent that other companies are diversifying their operations by moving into the drug field.

The Chief Economist of the Federal Trade Commission has testified that, on the basis of advice given by investment analysts, there is no reason to conclude that the drug industry is a uniquely risky industry. In fact, it appears that large drug companies should have little difficulty obtaining adequate capital for growth should they choose to go into the market for it. Actually, however, their earnings are large enough to preclude the frequent need for equity capital.

If new Federal regulations concerning drug safety, drug efficacy, and drug advertising have had any significant effect in reducing drug profits, this is not evident in recent drug company profit statements.

The "Reasonableness" of Drug Prices

Whether prescription drug prices set by the major manufacturers are "too high," "reasonable," or "too low" is obviously a problem which cannot be resolved to the mutual satisfaction of all manufacturers and all consumers.

It appears, however, that current drug prices at the manufacturer's level are marked by these characteristics:

- They reflect research and development costs which are relatively high in comparison with other industries, and which include a substantial degree of effort yielding only duplicative or "me-too" drugs and combination products that contribute little to the improvement of health care.
- They reflect promotion efforts which are high and are directed primarily to physicians.
- They reflect a high degree of competition based essentially on quality and innovation, rather than the normal competition based on quality, innovation, and price.

   We find, therefore, that the exceptionally high rate of profit which generally marks the drug industry is not accompanied by any peculiar degree of risk, or by any unique difficulties in obtaining growth capital, and that industry profits have not been significantly reduced by new governmental regulations concerning drug safety, drug efficacy, or drug advertising.

It is also evident from this study that there are certain problem areas which call for cooperative study and action by the drug industry, private groups, and the Federal Government.

Accordingly, the Task Force recommends that the Secretary of Health, Education, and Welfare should call one or more conferences with representatives of the drug industry, pharmacy, clinical medicine, and consumer groups to consider–

   a. Provision of incentives to the drug industry to invest more research effort in products representing significant improvements to therapy and less in duplicative, noncontributory drug products and combinations.

   b. Development of a registration and licensing system under which no drug product would be permitted in interstate commerce unless produced under quality control standards set by the Secretary of Health, Education, and Welfare.

   c. Limitation of free drug samples, by industry agreement or legislation, to those specifically requested by prescribers.

   d. Development of more effective methods for ascertaining actual acquisition costs of prescription drugs.

Similarly, it is evident that certain other areas of concern require detailed analysis by appropriate agencies of the Federal Government.

The Task Force therefore recommends that the Secretary of Health, Education, and Welfare should call for a joint study by the Department of Health, Education, and Welfare, the Department of Commerce, the Department of Justice, the Federal Trade Commission, and other Federal agencies to consider–

   a. The substantial differences in the prices at which drug products are offered to community pharmacies and to hospitals and government agencies.

   b. The substantial differences in the prices at which drug products are offered to American and foreign purchasers.

   c. Revision of patent and trademark laws on prescription drugs.

CHAPTER 3
THE DRUG DISTRIBUTORS

Between the manufacturers who make drugs and the patients who purchase them is a large, complex distribution network.

Included in this network are the major drug vendors–independent pharmacies, chain drugstores, prescription pharmacies, mail-order pharmacies, hospital pharmacies, dispensing physicians, and others. Considered with them in this section are the drug wholesalers.

Of the average prescription drug dollar paid by the consumer, about 50 cents is now taken by the manufacturer, 10 cents by the wholesaler, and 40 cents by the retailer.

On the basis of available data, it appears that profits before taxes for independent drugstores and other community pharmacies represent an average of about 5 percent of sales, or about 21 percent of net worth.

For hospital pharmacies, the average outpatient prescription price probably approximates the national community pharmacy average prescription price, even though drug costs and operating expenses may be appreciably lower, and no income taxes may be involved. Accordingly, the profit ratios for such hospital pharmacies may be substantially higher.

During the past three decades, the operations of the drug distribution system have undergone significant changes. For example, before World War II, most of the drug products handled were in bulk form, and were compounded into tablets, capsules, powders, solutions or other dosage forms by the pharmacist. Now about 95 percent are furnished by the manufacturer in final dosage form, ready for consumption.

Formerly, wholesalers handled the overwhelming proportion of drug products. Now, with manufacturers tending to sell directly to hospitals and the larger independent pharmacies and chains, the wholesalers handle only about 48 percent of the dollar volume of the market.

In the years to come, other changes in the number and nature of both wholesale and retail outlets will undoubtedly occur as the result of continuing economic pressures, health manpower shortages, the expansion of new types of careers in pharmacy, and the introduction of innovations enabling drug distributors to respond more effectively and efficiently to the health needs of patients.

A nationwide drug program under Medicare would inevitably provide new challenges and new opportunities. Certain aspects of such a program–notably the methods of reimbursement–deserve particular consideration.

Percentage Markup versus Dispensing Fee

Traditionally, most pharmacists have determined the retail price of a prescription drug by adding to the wholesale or acquisition cost a percentage of this cost–for example, 65 to 100 percent or more. Such a system is known as the percentage markup, or margin, method. This approach is currently supported by the National Association of Retail Druggists.

It is obvious that this method may serve as an inducement to a pharmacist to dispense the more expensive brand of a prescribed drug, if he has any choice in selecting the brand. To a considerable extent, it appears to lay a heavy burden upon the patient unfortunate enough to require expensive medication, and such an individual actually subsidizes the patient who requires less costly prescriptions.

More recently, some pharmacists have advocated the use of a dispensing fee which is the same regardless of the acquisition cost–an approach which has been endorsed particularly by the American Pharmaceutical Association. This method is based on the concept that dispensing activities represent a professional service that is generally unrelated to the acquisition cost of the drug, since the pharmacist usually performs the same service whether the medication costs 10 cents or $10.

As one authority has stated:

> "In applying the fee concept to a pharmacy practice, a pharmacist makes two assumptions which are the philosophic principles underlying its use. *First*, the pharmacist is a health specialist by virtue of his knowledge, education, and training, and dispensing prescription medication is a pharmaceutical service. For this act, he receives a fee . . . *Second*, the services a pharmacist provides in dispensing prescriptions is, in general, the same for all prescriptions, and the cost of providing this service remains relatively constant from one prescription to the next."

The use of the dispensing fee approach reduces the relative costs of high-priced medications, while increasing the costs of low-priced drugs, but the system appears to be more equitable since it eliminates the subsidization of some patients by others.

From the point of view of the vendor, employment of a fixed dispensing fee system means that physicians may attempt to help some of their patients needing long-term maintenance drugs by prescribing large quantities of drugs at one time, carrying only a single dispensing fee, rather than an original small prescription plus many small refills, each carrying a dispensing fee.

Dispensing Physicians

A dispensing physician is considered to be one who stocks a more-or-less complete line of drug products in his office, and sells these directly to his patient instead of writing a prescription for the patient to take to a pharmacy. The charges he makes may be essentially the same as those set by pharmacies in his community–or substantially higher or lower. (Not included in this category are physicians who administer a drug to a patient–usually in the course of a home or office visit–and include the cost as part of their fee for professional medical services.)

Some physicians find it necessary to sell drugs directly to patients in this way in emergencies, or because they practice in isolated areas in which no regular pharmacy services are available, but such situations would seem to be relatively uncommon.

In view of the acute shortage of physicians, the heavy demands already placed upon them to use the professional skills which only they possess, the possible conflict of interest which may be involved, and the propriety of burdening them with functions which can be performed at least as well by others, the Task Force believes that the role of dispensing physicians in an out-of-hospital drug program under Medicare warrants further study.

Government Pharmacies

It has been proposed that existing Veterans Administration and other Federal hospital pharmacies be used to dispense prescription drugs to beneficiaries of both the Medicare and Medicaid programs, either in person or by mail. Such an approach would presumably offer substantial savings, but the limited number and the location of these Federal hospital pharmacies would make it impractical for them in most cases to dispense except by mail, and would offer only limited pharmacist-patient relationships.

Physician-Owned Pharmacies

The ethical status of physician-owned pharmacies has recently been under consideration by the American Medical Association and other groups.

On the one hand, it has been held that such pharmacies offer particular convenience to patients, that they can often purchase drugs from manufacturers or wholesalers at prices which are not available to many community pharmacists, that they can maintain small inventories, and that they are more likely than community pharmacies to ensure that patients will receive the proper medication.

Although low inventories and relatively low acquisition costs could result in lower drug prices to patients, there is no evidence that the average prescription prices set by physician-owned pharmacies are any lower than those set by other pharmacies in the community. Further, there is no evidence that physician-owned pharmacies are any more or less likely to dispense improper medication.

In addition, it has been held that patients treated by a physician who both prescribes drugs and has a financial interest in the pharmacy which dispenses the drugs are clearly a captive audience, with no freedom of choice on where they will have their prescriptions filled. With the physician occupying a dual role as prescriber and dispenser, there is an obvious conflict of interest, with an evident risk of excessive prescribing. Further, a physician-dominated pharmacist may not exercise needed objective review of what may appear to him to be prescription errors.

Accordingly, the Task Force believes that the role of physician-owned pharmacies in any Medicare program warrants further study.

Physician-Owned Repackaging Companies

A drug-repackaging company is one which purchases a drug product from a manufacturer, usually in large quantities at a relatively low price, and then repackages it under its own brand name–and at its own price.

If such a firm is controlled by one or more physicians who set the price at an extraordinarily high level, and who prescribe its products under the repackaging company brand name–thus requiring the pharmacist to dispense it–the profits to the company and its prescriber-owners can be extraordinarily rewarding. Under these conditions, the cost to the patient can also be extraordinarily and needlessly high.

The conflict of interests and the potential exploitation of patients in such a situation are so apparent that the American Medical Association in 1967 declared it to be unethical.

Accordingly, the Task Force finds that products marketed by physician-owned repackaging companies should be considered unacceptable for reimbursement in any Medicare program except in those instances in which the Secretary of Health, Education, and Welfare determines that the availability of products marketed by such companies is in the public interest.

Prescription Price Information

There is an obvious need for patients to be able to determine readily the prices charged by the various pharmacies in their community. This appears to be particularly important in the case of long-term maintenance drugs.

The Task Force recognizes the difficulties in making such information easily available. Many patients are not told which drug has been prescribed for them–or are unable to decipher the physician's prescription. In many States, laws or regulations forbid pharmacies to advertise; even without such rules, however, advertising current prices on many thousands of different drugs and dosage forms would pose formidable practical problems. Physicians, especially those in large cities, are likely to be unaware of the different prices which may be set at different pharmacies.

We also recognize that the retail price of the prescription includes not only the cost of the ingredients, but also in some instances the availability of home delivery and 24-hour-a-day operations, as well as the professional services of the pharmacist–and that different pharmacists may wish to place different values on such services.

We recognize that many or most patients may wish to select a pharmacy more on the basis of convenient location than on the basis of price.

Nevertheless, if the patient is to maintain the right to select a pharmacy, he also has a right to know the prices it charges and to compare these with other prices.

We find there is a need for medical associations, pharmacy associations and consumer groups, working together at the local level, to develop mechanisms whereby patients may obtain information on local prescription prices, especially for long-term maintenance drugs.

Prescription Label Information

It is frequently necessary for a physician to determine the nature and amount of a prescription drug which a patient has been taking. In some instances–as in the case of a suspected adverse drug reaction, or accidental or deliberate overdose–the rapid identification of a drug may be a matter of life and death.

As a step in improving the quality of health care, the Task Force recommends that the Congress should enact legislation requiring that the containers of all dispensed prescription drugs be labeled with the identity, strength and quantity of the product, except where this is waived upon specific orders of the prescriber.

Prepackaging

Prepackage dispensing is now being utilized for a variety of drugs in Europe, and for such products as oral contraceptives in the United States. In certain cases, this technique appears to offer significant advantages.

To promote efficiency and minimize errors, the Task Force recommends that encouragement should be given to the wider use of prepackage dispensing, in which manufacturers prepare and pharmacists dispense tablets and capsules in precounted form, in sealed, prelabeled containers, and in such numbers as conform to those most frequently prescribed by physicians.

The New Role of Pharmacy

The pharmacy profession currently faces a dilemma which is partly though not entirely of its own making.

Many other aspects of health care–the practice of medicine and surgery, hospital operations, and particularly drug manufacture–have developed and adopted new devices and techniques which have remarkably improved the provision of health services. In contrast, the number of important new methods introduced to enhance the efficiency of retail pharmacy operations, at least during the past two or three decades, has not been noteworthy.

The Task Force recommends that the National Center for Health Services Research and Development should develop and support research to improve the efficiency and effectiveness of community and hospital pharmacy operations.

The role of the pharmacist is viewed by many people as simply transferring pills from a large bottle to a small one–counting tablets, typing labels, and calculating the price. Much of his time is seen as devoted to routine merchandising of cosmetics, shaving supplies, stationery and other commodities which have little or no relationship to health care.

This has raised doubts concerning the relevance of modern pharmacy education. As with other members of health professions, on the one hand, it would seem that much of the traditional education is not utilized, since a nonprofessional pharmacist–working under the supervision of a licensed pharmacist–can effectively perform many of the routine tasks of counting, labeling, and pricing. At the same time, many pharmacists are seeking a new role as a drug information specialist, and thus it would appear that their formal education has not taken this into account.

These problems regarding what the role of the pharmacist properly is–or should be–deserve careful consideration.

Pharmacist Aides

Experience in numerous pharmacies–military and nonmilitary Federal installations, nongovernmental hospitals, and others–has demonstrated that individuals without formal pharmacy education can effectively undertake many of the routine activities of pharmacists, under the supervision of a licensed pharmacist.

Such activities offer the possibility of developing the career of pharmacist aide, comparable to the nursing aide, the orthopedic aide, the pediatric aide, the obstetrical aide, and similar paramedical positions.

Drug Information Specialists

At the other end of the spectrum, it is also becoming evident that appropriately trained pharmacists may become new and vital members of the total health team by serving as drug information specialists.

Some community pharmacists are already providing such services. They do not prescribe, but they discuss practical details of drug administration, possible side-effects, and other facets of drug use with each patient to whom a prescription drug is dispensed. They maintain patient or family records which contain data on drugs which have been dispensed to each patient, allergic responses, and adverse reactions. They call to the attention of the physician any prescriptions which may have been written for the same patient by other physicians, and they refer to him any prescriptions which may involve drug-interaction, synergism, or similar effects.

Some hospitals–especially teaching institutions and those in major medical center complexes–are already using pharmacists as consultants on drug therapy. They serve not only as drug distributors, but also as sources of drug data for physicians, interns, residents, and nurses. They may participate in ward rounds with the staff, providing valuable drug information on both old and new drug products. Although they do not prescribe for patients, they enable the physicians who do prescribe to keep up more effectively with drug information.

While some pharmacists are already serving as drug information specialists, and others are probably competent to do so, not all pharmacists have adequate competency in this field. Some licensed pharmacists have received five or even six years of formal college training, but about 15 percent of those now in practice have received two years or less of formal pharmacy education, and nearly half of these have had courses lasting only about six months.

Pharmacy Education

The introduction of out-of-hospital prescription drug program under Medicare, with the probability of a very large increase in drug utilization, coming at a time when quality of health care, costs, and shortages in health manpower are all matters of great national concern, would present pharmacy with probably the most critical challenge it has faced in half a century.

The manner in which pharmacists, pharmacy associations, pharmacy schools, and the pertinent State pharmacy agencies respond to increasing demands for pharmaceutical services will unquestionably determine in large measure how the pharmacy profession will evolve during the years to come.

The Task Force commends the efforts of those pharmacy schools and State pharmacy associations which are already stressing continuing postgraduate education.

As a guide to additional responses which should be made, there is a clear need for a broad study of pharmacy education at all levels.

> **The Task Force therefore recommends that the Bureau of Health Manpower should support–**
>
> **a. The development of a pharmacist aide curriculum in junior colleges and other educational institutions.**

> ***b. The development of appropriate curricula in medical and pharmacy schools for training pharmacists to serve as drug information specialists on the health team.***
>
> ***c. A broad study of present and future requirements in pharmacy, adequacy of current pharmacy education, and the educational changes which must be made.***

Pharmacy Laws

The present patchwork of State pharmacy laws, regulations, and codes of ethics obviously reflects attempts to cope with a variety of pharmacy problems on a piecemeal basis. Whether they are aimed at the protection of the public health or the prevention of competition–fair or unfair–it is not clear in all cases.

Many of these rules seem to have derived from periods of manpower excesses. They block efforts to cope with the present shortages of skilled manpower, the need for mobility to meet rapidly changing health needs, and the probable development of new careers in pharmacy.

> ***The Task Force recommends that the Health Services and Mental Health Administration should support studies of State laws, regulations, and codes, with priority given to the establishment of model State licensing laws, uniform reciprocity standards, and provisions for the utilization of pharmacy aides.***

CHAPTER 4
THE DRUG PRESCRIBERS

In the modern use of drugs, important roles are played by the drug researcher, the manufacturer, the distributor, the pharmacist, and the official who carries the legal responsibility for drug safety, efficacy and quality. But the most strategic role is that of the physician who prescribes the drug.

It is the physician who has major responsibility for the welfare of the patient.

It is the physician who is constantly faced with an awesome assortment of competitive and often duplicative products.

It is the physician who is the target of a barrage of advice, information, guidance, and promotion from detail men, advertisements, medical articles, pamphlets, bulletins, and throw-away journals.

And it is the physician who–with or without adequate training and competent advice–must make the decision on which drug or drugs to prescribe.

On his decision may well depend the health or even the life of his patient. On it will depend, at least in part, the quality, cost and effectiveness of any drug insurance program, governmental or nongovernmental. And on it will depend the economic well-being of a drug company.

Rational Prescribing

The appropriate selection of a drug–the right drug for the right patient, in the right amounts at the right times–is generally defined as rational prescribing, and any significant deviation is considered to be irrational prescribing.

Rational prescribing is obviously the result of judgments on many points–the safety and efficacy of the drug for the clinical problem at hand, the advantages or disadvantages of alternative forms of therapy, the most appropriate dosage form, the length and intensity of treatment, the possible side-effects or adverse reactions, and the possibility of drug interaction.

To these may be added judgments concerning relative costs.

Rational prescribing is clearly a major goal for the welfare of patients. It is likewise a major goal for any drug insurance program. Here, emphasis has been placed not directly on achieving rational prescribing but rather on preventing some of the more serious or costly forms of irrational prescribing. Among the latter are these:

- The use of drugs without demonstrated efficacy.
- The use of drugs with an inherent hazard not justified by the seriousness of the illness.
- The use of drugs in excessive amounts, or for excessive periods of time, or inadequate amounts for inadequate periods.
- The use of a costly duplicative or "me-too" product when an equally effective but less expensive drug is available.
- The use of a costly combination product when equally effective but less expensive drugs are available individually.
- The simultaneous use of two or more drugs without appropriate consideration of their possible interaction.
- Multiple prescribing, by one or several physicians for the same patient, of drugs which may be unnecessary, cumulative, interacting, or needlessly expensive.

We recognize that some patients may be receiving as many as 16 to 20 different drugs simultaneously, prescribed by either one or several different physicians, and that often physicians may not be aware that their patients are receiving drugs prescribed by others.

We see no reason to believe that any or all of these types of irrational prescribing can be effectively prevented–or that rational prescribing can be effectively induced–merely by rules and regulations. Instead, we believe the objective of rational prescribing can be reached most effectively through improving medical education–particularly in the area of clinical pharmacology–at both the undergraduate and postgraduate levels, supplying practicing physicians with objective data on which they can base their individual prescribing decisions, and supporting those in hospitals, clinics, medical societies and health insurance programs who are seeking to achieve rational prescribing by their fellow practitioners.

The Teaching of Pharmacology

In most American medical schools, the principal course in pharmacology is given during the second year. Generally, this is the only formal exposure of the student to the subject.

The nature of pharmacology instruction has been a matter of much debate but little change. Although it is in reality a clinical as well as a basic science, it is taught primarily as a basic subject, with emphasis on the principles of drug action, a review of specific drug groups, examples of drug applications, and the broad fundamentals of prescription writing.

After the usual course in basic pharmacology, most medical students are given no formal training in the applied aspects of this field–in clinical pharmacology–but left to acquire what practical training they can absorb from a variety of courses in the several fields of clinical medicine.

Perhaps the most serious criticism of this informal exposure is that it fails to equip the soon-to-be physician with the essential scientific and critical attitudes towards the use of drugs and the evaluation of drug promotion–probably the most intensive promotion to which he will be subjected for the rest of his professional career.

The Task Force has noted that some medical schools have responded to such a deficiency by establishing courses in clinical pharmacology or pharmacotherapeutics. In these courses dealing with the practical aspects of drug prescribing, emphasis is generally placed on such subjects as the design of comparative clinical drug trials, and the techniques of statistical analysis. Also included in some courses is the evaluation of drug advertising and promotional material, and the importance of drug costs.

Many who participate in these and related programs have received a major part of their training in the Section of Clinical Pharmacology in the National Heart Institute of the National Institutes of Health.

> ***The Task Force recommends that the Department of Health, Education, and Welfare should provide expanded support to medical schools, enabling them to include a course in clinical pharmacology as an integral part of the medical curriculum.***

Postgraduate Education

Upon entering private practice, the average physician, knowingly or unknowingly, becomes the key figure in drug marketing strategy.

- He must choose from a very large number of competitive and often duplicative products.
- He must deal with a very large amount of advice, biased or unbiased, from detail men, advertisements and other forms of promotion.
- Substantial efforts are made on his behalf by the drug industry and others to prevent any interference with his right to prescribe as he sees fit.
- Finally, it is assumed that he has the training, experience, and time to weigh the claims and available evidence, and thus to make the proper selection.

Everything, of course, hinges on the validity of this final assumption.

> ***We find that few practicing physicians seem inclined to voice any question of their competency in this field of therapeutic judgments. We also find, however, that the ability of an individual physician to make sound judgments under quite confusing conditions is now a matter of serious concern to leading clinicians, scientists, and medical educators.***

A distinguished pharmacologist, for example, has stated that lack of knowledge and sophistication in the proper use of drugs is perhaps the greatest deficiency of the average physician today. Other medical leaders have pointed to the wide discrepancy in the prescribing habits of the average physician as compared to the prescribing methods recommended by panels of medical experts. Still others have commented on the continued use by the average physician of products which have been found unnecessary or unacceptable by specially qualified therapeutics committees in hospitals and clinics.

We note that the most widely used source of prescribing information is essentially a compilation of the most widely advertised drugs.

The responsibility for these and other deficiencies has been placed on various factors:

- Inadequate training in the clinical application of drug knowledge during the undergraduate medical curriculum.
- Inadequate sources of objective information on both drug properties and drug costs.
- Widespread reliance by prescribers for their continuing education upon the promotional materials distributed by drug manufacturers.
- The exceedingly rapid rate of introduction and obsolescence of prescription drug specialties.
- The limited time available to practicing physicians to examine, evaluate, and maintain currency with the claims for both old drugs and newly marketed products.
- The constant insistence on the idea that the average physician, without guidance from expert colleagues, does in fact possess the necessary ability to make scientifically sound judgments in this complicated field.

Information Sources

Several significant approaches have been attempted to cope with this problem. In the United States, a small number of independent publications–which do not publish advertising–seek to present objective evaluations of the efficacy, safety, rationality, and occasionally the costs of specific drugs. These have relatively limited circulation, but are highly esteemed by medical leaders.

Many American hospitals and clinics utilize pharmacy and therapeutics committees to develop formularies which serve as guidelines to the staff members of the institutions. These, too, appear to contribute significantly to rational prescribing.

Other approaches to the problem of communicating objective and updated drug information have been proposed. These include closed-circuit television programs originating in medical centers; the development of community pharmacy and therapeutics committees; the utilization of existing regional medical programs to sponsor continuing drug information programs; and the use of hospital pharmacies as drug information centers.

Several foreign drug programs–notably those in Great Britain, Australia, and New Zealand–provide all physicians with prescribing guidelines prepared by panels of independent medical experts. Such publications–frequently updated to meet changing conditions–have been widely accepted by the medical profession in those countries.

In the United States, much useful information on such factors as indications, contraindications, dosages, toxicity, and side effects is included in the so-called package inserts which must be enclosed with each container of drugs. While these are of considerable value, they are not seen often enough by the practicing physician to be of practical aid in prescribing.

From the foregoing, it is evident that many and perhaps most American physicians do not have adequate access to complete and objective information on prescription drugs. The existing compilations of data do not generally touch on relative costs, and they do not offer the ready comparison of generic-name products and their brand-name counterparts which would facilitate the rational and economic prescribing of drugs.

> ***In consideration of these factors, in view of the unfilled informational needs evident in this country, and as a major contribution to improving the quality of health care, the Task Force recommends that the Department of Health, Education, and Welfare should establish or support a publication providing objective, up-to-date information and guidelines on drug therapy, based on the expert advice of the medical community.***

> ***We recommend that the Department of Health, Education, and Welfare should support the efforts of county medical societies, pharmacy and therapeutics committees, medical foundations, and medical schools in taking the responsibility for providing continuing education to physicians on rational prescribing.***

The Bureau of Health Manpower, the Division of Regional Medical Programs, and the National Library of Medicine in particular should assign high priority to the support of such efforts.

Finally, we recommend that the Secretary of Health, Education, and Welfare should be authorized to publish and distribute to all physicians, pharmacies, hospitals and other appropriate individuals and institutions a drug compendium listing all lawfully available prescription drugs, including such information as available dosage forms, clinical effects, indications and contraindications for use, and methods of administration, together with price information on each listed product, in readily accessible and comprehensive form.

CHAPTER 5
CURRENT AMERICAN AND FOREIGN PROGRAMS

The provision of out-of-hospital prescription drugs through governmental or private insurance programs has been undertaken in one form or another for nearly a century. Many of these include techniques and approaches which deserve consideration in any out-of-hospital program that might be designed under Medicare.

Accordingly, the Task Force has examined a wide variety of ongoing programs–all of the major drug programs conducted by the Federal Government, a number of selected State programs, six of the leading private programs in this country, and the major programs in eleven foreign countries.

These programs are not directly comparable. In some foreign countries, for example, national economic and social structures lend themselves to controls and methods of operation which are probably not suitable in the United States. Certain aspects of military drug programs may not be adaptable for civilian programs. Other approaches utilized in private programs may be impractical for a government operation.

Nevertheless, a study of these diverse systems has proved to be illuminating. It has clearly indicated that out-of-hospital prescription drugs can be provided under programs that are medically acceptable and economically sound.

Federal Programs

Through direct purchasing or reimbursement, the Federal Government is now concerned with the provision of prescription drugs through several major programs. As shown in Table 2, expenditures for drugs in these programs totaled about $514 million in fiscal year 1967.

DOD Military Procurement. The largest direct drug procurement program is that of the Department of Defense, with its responsibility for supplying about 3,000 military establishments in this country and overseas. A major characteristic of the DOD operation is its testing and inspection program to assure drug quality and the ability of the products to withstand prolonged exposure to climatic extremes. DOD sets its own drug specifications, maintains its own manufacturing plant inspectors, and operates its own testing program. Manufacturers must undergo stringent pre-award surveys of their facilities as well as testing of their products in DOD laboratories. After drug contracts are

TABLE 2. Estimated Federal Expenditures for Prescription Drugs, Fiscal Year 1967.

	(Millions)
Direct Purchase	
Department of Defense	[a] $111.0
Public Health Service	[b] 4.1
Veterans Administration	[c] 39.5
Federal Supply Schedule Contracts	[d] 6.2
Total Direct	160.8
Reimbursement Programs	
CHAMPUS	0.2
VA Hometown Pharmacies	2.9
Public Health Service	0.7
Medicare In-Hospital	[e] 230.0
Medicaid	[f] 119.4
Total Reimbursement	353.2
Total, Federal Drug Expenditures	514.0

[a] Includes $92.4 million purchased through Defense Supply Center, Philadelphia, Pa., and approximately $15.7 million purchased through Federal Supply Schedule Contracts; remainder purchased locally.
[b] Includes $1.3 million purchased through PHS Supply Service Center, Perry Point, Md., and $2.8 million from other sources including the Veterans Administration.
[c] Includes $14.6 million purchased through Federal Supply Schedule contracts administered by VA for General Services Administration.
[d] Includes purchases for miscellaneous Federal agencies.
[e] Includes $115.0 million for overhead drug expenses of hospitals and extended care facilities.
[f] Includes other Federally-supported State Public Assistance Programs; excludes $105.9 million, which was the State portion of the total drug program expenses.

awarded, both the plant facilities and the stored products are continuously spot-checked, and DOD actively solicits reports from military hospitals and physicians on drug quality, therapeutic efficacy, and adverse reactions.

About 240 of the 1,200 drugs currently stocked are purchased under generic name.

The DOD policy is to purchase drugs under contract from the lowest "responsible bidder." It may buy foreign-made drugs where the acquisition cost is at least 50 percent less than "responsible" domestic bids. The same pre-award standards and continuing surveillance imposed on domestic firms are applied to foreign manufacturers with DOD contracts.

As a Federal purchasing agency, DOD may purchase patented products from unlicensed manufacturers.

DOD Military Medicare. Through its Civilian Health and Medical Program of the Uniformed Services (CHAMPUS), the Department of Defense provides out-of-hospital prescription drugs through hometown pharmacies to some 6.5 million eligible retired military personnel and military dependents. Various carriers are used for program administration.

Any pharmacy willing to meet CHAMPUS requirements may participate. The pharmacist is reimbursed for the acquisition cost of the drug plus a dispensing fee which has been set for each State.

Each eligible beneficiary must first meet a deductible requirement of $50 per year–or $100 per year per family–and pay a co-insurance charge of 20 or 25 percent, depending on beneficiary status.

No formulary requirements are involved.

The average prescription price in 1967 was reported to be about $4.15.

Veterans Administration. In 1967, the VA purchased drugs and biologicals costing $39.5 million for use in its own hospitals and pharmacies, and also procured drugs for other Federal agencies, such as the Public Health Service and the Office of Economic Opportunity.

Of the drugs used in VA pharmacies, about 86 percent are purchased from some 250 manufacturers who have been approved by on-site inspections. Each VA hospital has its own drug formulary of about 700 to 2,000 items developed by its own pharmacy and therapeutics committee, and tailored to fit the needs of the institution. The formularies are used as guidelines rather than prescribing limitations, since non-formulary drugs may also be prescribed.

Chemical equivalent drugs are widely used where available.

In addition, the VA Hometown Pharmacy Program provides out-of-hospital prescription drugs to eligible beneficiaries, generally those with service-connected disabilities. The hometown program, which involved an expenditure of $2.7 million in 1967, provides for reimbursement to pharmacies on the basis of acquisition cost plus a dispensing fee. No formulary is used in this program, and no deductible or co-payment is required.

Office of Economic Opportunity. Through its neighborhood Health Centers, OEO provides pharmaceutical services for about 800,000 persons in 44 programs.

Eligibility requirements vary but generally are based on a "poverty line" schedule, on Medicaid standards, or on other guidelines established by the community. Each center makes its own determination about the use of a formulary. No deductible or co-payment is required.

Several of the centers provide direct drug services in their own pharmacies, while the others provide for reimbursement to community pharmacies on the basis of acquisition cost plus a dispensing fee.

Public Health Service. In 1967, PHS expended more than $4 million for drugs for its own operations, and also purchased drugs for Civil Defense stockpiling.

Of the drugs procured for PHS activities, some were used by the National Institutes of Health and the National Institute of Mental Health, but most were dispensed through the Division of Direct Health Services–with 11 hospital and 14 clinic pharmacies–and the Division of Indian Health. The latter operates 51 hospitals with pharmacies, and contracts with about 200 community pharmacies that furnish prescription drugs to Indian beneficiaries.

Each PHS hospital has its own formulary, but exceptions are made for the provision of non-formulary drugs. Physicians who contract with PHS are not obliged to use the formularies.

Pharmacies participating under contract with the Division of Indian Health are required to dispense the least expensive drug products they have in stock which will meet the physician's requirements when a generic prescription is written. The price may not exceed the price to the general public.

No deductibles or co-insurance requirements are involved in any of the PHS out-of-hospital programs.

Medicare. Data from the Medicare program relating to the cost of drugs provided to beneficiaries in hospitals and extended care facilities are not yet available. However, on the basis of recent studies of drug use in hospitals in general, it is estimated that in fiscal 1967 roughly $230 million was spent under Medicare for drugs, with about half of this amount representing product cost and the remainder the cost of dispensing and administration (see Table 2).

Under Medicare, in-hospital drugs must be listed in one of several official compendia or in a formulary established by the hospital's pharmacy and therapeutics committee. Medicare requires that drug charges to the government must be "reasonable."

Public Assistance. Under Medicaid and other public assistance programs with joint Federal-State support, an estimated $225.3 million was spent for prescription drugs in fiscal 1967, of which an estimated $119.4 million was paid by the Federal Government (Table 2). Federal-State vendor payments of $225.3 million (including about $43 million for in-hospital drugs) represented 9.6 percent of all medical care services provided in that year, and were made to hospitals, pharmacists, and other licensed vendors.

The Federal share of payments to vendors for drugs and drug services ranged from 50 to 83 percent, depending on the nature and extent of the program in each State, with an average of about 53 percent.

In such programs, no deductibles or co-payments are generally involved, although one non-Medicaid State program included a co-payment requirement but provided funds to the recipients to cover such payments.

Further details on these public assistance programs are presented in the following section.

State Programs

Vendor drug programs for recipients of Medicaid and other public assistance funds are now operating in 38 States and Territories. The range in their utilization, costs, and benefits is very large.

Thus, among all eligible beneficiaries, the utilization rates in 1967 ranged from 26 percent in Missouri and Tennessee to 91 percent in New Hampshire and 99 percent in Rhode Island.

The average annual number of prescriptions per user ranged from about 10 in New Mexico to 46 in Indiana.

The average annual expenditure per user ranged from $39.35 in New Jersey to $148.95 in Florida, $155.67 in Nebraska, and $158.58 in Indiana.

The average cost per prescription ranged from $2.91 in Kentucky and $2.94 in Illinois to $4.74 in New Mexico.

Because of the diversity and complexity of the various State drug programs, the Task Force selected five for intensive study–California, because of its size; Louisiana and West Virginia, because of their approach in approving drugs used only for the treatment of specific diseases; Kentucky, because of its limited formulary; and Pennsylvania, because of its extensive formulary, which is used primarily as a guide to prescribing.

Other studies were conducted on the programs in Indiana, Nebraska, North Carolina, Oklahoma, and South Dakota.

In nearly all of these States, per capita drug costs and average prescription prices for program beneficiaries were higher than those for the total public. Whether this was the result of program abuse or of the greater health needs of those receiving public assistance cannot be readily determined.

There was no consistent pattern of vendor payments, with some states reimbursing on the basis of customary and usual charges, some on acquisition cost plus a percentage markup, some on acquisition cost plus a dispensing fee, and some using a combination of percentage markup plus dispensing fee. Several set dollar limits. There was no clearcut relationship between any of these methods and program costs.

Where acquisition cost was a factor in the reimbursing formula, this was generally presumed to be the listed wholesale price, although it is understood that this list price has little if any relationship to the actual acquisition cost. Few States made any efforts through spot audits to determine actual acquisition cost.

Administrative expenses have been estimated to average about 50 cents per prescription, with the lowest cost–about 20 cents–reported in Louisiana. Differences in estimating administrative costs, however, make it impossible to make exact comparisons.

Among the States studied, none was applying data processing techniques to the extent necessary for effective utilization review.

Only one State–North Carolina–had tested the effect of a deterrent charge to the patient. In February 1967, North Carolina required the recipient to pay the first dollar of the cost of each prescription, and at the same time provided beneficiaries with monthly cash payments from which to pay medical expenses. Within about two months, although the number of prescriptions actually increased, the total cost of the prescription drug program was reduced.

While there seemed to be wide agreement among officials of many States that such a co-payment requirement would probably be a highly effective method of cost control, there was no such agreement on the effect of this technique in limiting the access of welfare beneficiaries to the health care they required.

The influence of limited formularies alone also appears to be questionable. Although the use of a highly restrictive formulary is associated in several States with effective cost control, such control also has been noted in Pennsylvania, with a virtually unlimited formulary but with restrictions on quantity and number of refills.

Many States urged or required the dispensing of low-cost chemical equivalent products where available. Under such conditions, no significant instances of lack of clinical equivalency were reported.

We find, therefore, that in Medicaid and other State public assistance programs, no single method will by itself guarantee program efficiency, but without at least two features–reasonable formulary restrictions and effective data processing procedures–program controls will be ineffective. Although a co-payment requirement may not be widely acceptable in public assistance drug programs, its value in controlling costs in other programs seems evident.

Private Programs

Several nongovernmental programs to provide prescription drugs to members of unions and other groups have been in operation in this country for many decades, and others have been developed in more recent years.

For special examination, the Task Force selected six of these– Prepaid Prescription Plans, Inc.; Paid Prescriptions, Inc.; United Mine Workers; the Kaiser Foundation Health Plan; Group Health Cooperative of Puget Sound; and the new Blue Cross plan.

As in the case of State programs, these private programs offered a variety of approaches. Some utilized their own pharmacies. Several used restrictive formularies, while others reimbursed for any prescribed product.

All were financed through monthly dues or premiums.

Major economies in these private plans were found associated with the use of formularies, frequent field audits to determine actual acquisition costs by vendors, and the use of a co-payment or similar requirement. The greatest economies were noted in those programs in which the institution served as the purchaser of the drug products, rather than as a reimburser, and thus could obtain competitive or negotiated bids.

Several of the programs included in this study either urged or required the use of available low-cost chemical equivalents. No significant problems with lack of clinical equivalency were reported.

Foreign Programs

The greatest experience with prescription drug programs has been achieved in a number of foreign countries. Fifteen of them in eleven nations were selected by the Task Force for special study–Australia, Belgium, Denmark, France, Great Britain, The Netherlands, New Zealand, Norway, Sweden, West Germany, and the provincial programs of Alberta, British Columbia, Manitoba, Ontario, and Saskatchewan in Canada. Less intensive studies were conducted on the programs in Italy and Switzerland.

All of these nations show wide variations in demographic characteristics, government operations, industrial development, social philosophy, local tradition, and even medical tradition, and certain portions of their health insurance programs may not be suitable for use in the United States. Nevertheless, most of the procedures considered for prescription drug insurance programs in this country have already been tried in one form or another in these foreign programs.

In all of the countries included in the Task Force study–which represent nearly all of the major prescription drug programs in the world–the program is financed by employee or employer contributions, or by voluntary or compulsory participation in various "sickness funds" and insurance plans.

Some, including several of the Canadian programs, are designed exclusively for public assistance beneficiaries. Others cover the entire population, regardless of economic status, while still others have programs providing one set of benefits to welfare beneficiaries or pensioners, and another set to those who are not public assistance recipients.

Most of the prescription drug programs, especially in Europe, are integral parts of national health insurance systems.

In most countries for which statistical data are available, it is evident that there has been a steady increase in the average number of prescriptions per year, in the average prescription cost, and in the cost of the entire program. The prices of specific drug products and of average prescriptions are generally lower than those in the United States; these differences appear to reflect lower labor costs, lower purchasing power, and similar factors, and also more intense price competition among drug manufacturers.

In nearly all countries surveyed in this study, a formulary of one type or another is used to improve rational prescribing, ensure drug quality, and control costs. In most, but not all cases, there are provisions for prescribing an unlisted drug when this is clinically indicated.

The drug lists of Norway, Sweden and Denmark are structured to provide only essential drugs for serious diseases. In France, Great Britain and West Germany, formularies are essentially unlimited, and in the last two countries are noncompulsory; all three of these countries, however, are currently considering the use of more restrictive formularies.

In Australia and New Zealand, and in several European countries, formularies have proved to be highly effective in controlling costs. The Australian government, for example, has no authority to set prices for drugs but uses inclusion in the formulary as an indirect means of price control–that is, if the price is considered too high in relation to its therapeutic advantages by a committee of medical advisors, a drug may not be included in the list. New Zealand negotiates prices, but will pay only at the level established for an acceptable chemical equivalent where one is available. Most of the countries have either established maximum retail prices or negotiated price agreements with manufacturers.

Compulsory licensing of patents is provided by law in most of the countries, but the law is seldom invoked. It may be used if the manufacturer of an "essential" or "necessary" drug refuses to reduce its price to what the health program considers to be a reasonable level.

With the exception of France, all countries in this group reimburse the drug vendor rather than the patient. The price paid to the vendor is usually determined on the basis of acquisition cost plus an established percentage markup, a dispensing fee, a container fee, or a combination of any of these. In The Netherlands, a capitation system is used in which the patient is required to have his prescription filled at a single pharmacy, and the pharmacist is paid a per capita fee for each patient registered with him.

In several countries, drug utilization review is provided through central or local boards or committees of physicians. In New Zealand, for example, medical representatives visit physicians to discuss drugs, local prescribing patterns and any individual prescribing habits which might seem to represent irrational prescribing. In Australia and Great Britain, these visits occur when the individual physician's prescribing pattern appears to represent unusually high costs.

Nearly all of these countries recommend or require the use of low-cost chemical equivalents where available. No significant problems with lack of clinical equivalency have been reported. Controversy over generic-name prescribing in Australia, New Zealand and most of the European countries studied by the Task Force has not reached the heights noted in the United States.

Quality control in many of the countries is achieved by registration of all drugs sold in the country, as well as by various types of drug testing. Often a drug evaluation committee or commission composed of physicians, pharmacists, and drug industry representatives has the responsibility for determining which drugs will be registered and which tests will be imposed. Testing varies from batch analysis to complete laboratory research of the formulation and its possible side effects.

Some programs call for patient participation through a fixed co-payment or percentage co-insurance. The effect of such a requirement was demonstrated in Great Britain, when the co-payment requirement was abolished and program costs promptly rose substantially.

*   *   *

From a survey of the major governmental and private prescription drug programs in the United States and foreign countries, the Task Force finds that–

> ***Establishment of an out-of-hospital prescription drug program for the elderly or for other population groups has been shown to be economically feasible in many countries.***

> ***Rational prescribing, with due regard to quality of health care as well as to program costs, can be improved through the cooperation of physicians, pharmacists, drug manufacturers, and a governmental agency.***

Reasonable program costs appear to be associated with (a) the use of a formulary developed by or in cooperation with the medical community, (b) the use of co-payment or co-insurance, (c) the use of utilization review procedures to prevent or minimize irrational prescribing, (d) the use of appropriate electronic or other data processing methods, with appropriate drug coding techniques, (e) simplified determination of beneficiary eligibility, (f) population coverage which obviates the adverse selection of high-risk beneficiaries, (g) the use of a vendor payment formula based on actual acquisition cost verified by field audits rather than any catalog or wholesale list price, and (h) operation with the program serving as the legal purchasing agency, with utilization of competitive and negotiated bids, rather than merely as the reimbursing agency.

*   *   *

From its consideration of ongoing prescription drug programs, the Task Force finds that a permanent mechanism is needed at the Federal level to collect, analyze and exchange information, and to provide effective coordination of drug-related activities among the agencies involved.

We therefore recommend that the Federal Interdepartmental Health Policy Council should concern itself with the coordination of all ongoing Federal prescription drug purchase and reimbursement programs.

We recommend that a special subcommittee of the Council should be appointed for this purpose.

CHAPTER 6
DRUG QUALITY

Intimately related to the costs of drugs in any insurance program is the quality of those products. Involved here is not only the financial soundness of the program; more significant is the quality of health care which is being provided.

During the past eighteen months, the Task Force has considered various aspects of drug quality, and reported on a number of significant developments:

- Programs undertaken to evaluate the adequacy of existing drug standards and to institute changes in those standards necessary to assure the clinical equivalency of chemically equivalent drugs.
- Steps taken by the Food and Drug Administration to strengthen the enforcement of its regulations concerning Good Manufacturing Practices.
- The review of the efficacy of some 2,900 drugs first marketed between 1938 and 1962 which have been under examination by the National Academy of Sciences/National Research Council.
- The successful drug quality control program of two of the Government's major drug-purchasing agencies, the Department of Defense and the Public Health Service, as well as those of several foreign nations.
- A special study instituted by the Task Force for the objective determination of the biological equivalency of selected chemical equivalents. (This study is described in a following section.)

Despite budgetary restraints and the need to develop new methodology, steady progress has been made in all of these areas.

Clinical Equivalency

During the past several years, the clinical equivalency of generic-name products has been the center of particularly heated controversy.

This issue may be presented as follows:

> *Given two drug products containing essentially the same amount of the same active ingredient in the same dosage form–that is, two chemical equivalents–will they produce essentially the same clinical effects?*

This question, of increasing interest to both physicians and patients, is now under careful consideration by the scientific community. Objective research has shown that in certain instances the clinical effects may not be the same.

> **The Task Force finds, however, that on the basis of available evidence, lack of clinical equivalency among chemical equivalents meeting all official standards has been grossly exaggerated as a major hazard to the public health.**

Where low-cost chemical equivalents have been employed–in foreign drug programs, in leading American hospitals, in State welfare programs, in Veterans Administration and Public Health Service hospitals, and in American military operations–instances of clinical nonequivalency have seldom been reported, and few of these have had significant therapeutic consequences.

Even though such cases are few, and others may well be reported in the future, these cannot be ignored, and the problem deserves careful consideration because of the medical and economic policies which are involved.

The interrelation of medical and economic factors is especially obvious in the case of two chemically equivalent products, both containing the same amount of the active ingredient and both meeting legal standards, but priced at different levels.

If the physician can be given reasonable assurance that two such competitive products will, in fact, give predictably equivalent clinical effects, then his choice between the two may well be based on relative costs. Under such conditions, there would be little justification for prescribing a relatively expensive brand of a drug when an equally effective counterpart is available at substantially lower cost. Similarly, there would be little justification for a Federal drug program to provide for reimbursement of such an expensive brand.

But if the physician cannot be given this assurance, his clinical judgment would dictate that he use only the product which can be expected to yield the desired clinical effects–regardless of cost or any other nonmedical factor.

The physician should be given assurance–not in the form of advertising, promotion, or the established image of the manufacturer involved, but in the form of objective, scientific data. In view of the thousands of drug products on the market, the accumulation of such data might seem to be monumental. But, with the exception of a few drugs for which adequate analytical methods are currently unknown, the Task Force has noted that the problem is by no means insoluble.

Clinical Equivalency and Biological Equivalency

For the direct determination of *clinical equivalency*, it would be necessary to compare drug products containing the same active ingredient, in the same tablet or capsule or other dosage form, in the same amounts, and measurement of their relative effects in human patients in the alleviation of symptoms or the control of a specific disease.

Except perhaps in rare instances, such a comparison appears to be impractical at this time. It would be time consuming and costly. It would be complicated not only by individual human differences but by differences in the symptoms or diseases under consideration.

Clinical equivalency studies could be conducted in experimental animals, but the nature of specific diseases and the nature of drug absorption and action in animals and human beings may not be directly comparable in all cases.

Instead, attention has been directed to the use of *biological equivalency*-or relative biological or physiological availability-measured in normal subjects as a proxy for the direct measurement and comparison of therapeutic effects.

This is based on the general agreement among pharmacologists that with most drugs-certainly those taken orally for their effect on internal tissues and organs-their therapeutic effectiveness will be closely related to the absorption of the active ingredient into the blood stream.

Thus, it is assumed that if the active ingredient in two or more chemically equivalent products reaches the blood (or other fluid or tissue)-and becomes biologically or physiologically available-at the same time and in the same amounts, their therapeutic effects will be essentially the same.

Among the formulation factors which may be involved here, and involved in any possible nonequivalency of orally-ingested products, are particle size; crystal form; the pressures and other conditions used in tabletmaking; and adjuvants, such as substances incorporated as fillers, lubricants, binders, coatings, flavorings, colorings, and tablet-disintegrating agents.

Attention has also been directed toward physicochemical tests which might be used to indicate biological equivalency. Perhaps the most important of these is the dissolution rate. Once a drug is dissolved in the gastrointestinal fluid, absorption is usually rapid. It is not surprising, therefore, that reported instances of clinical nonequivalency are rare among drugs which are highly soluble or administered in solution but most frequent among drugs of inherently low solubility which are administered in solid dosage forms such as tablets and capsules.

Biological Equivalency Trials

In consideration of the foregoing, the Task Force initiated a program in the fall of 1967 to determine scientifically the biological equivalency of a number of chemical equivalents.

A major phase of the investigation was an attempt to determine whether any observed differences in biological equivalency could be related to differences in the physical or chemical characteristics of the products.

It was recognized at the outset that such trials were urgently needed for relatively few drugs. For example, among the 409 products most widely used by the elderly–and which accounted for about 88 percent of all prescription drugs dispensed to this group, there were only 86 which were dispensed under brand name but could have been dispensed under generic name from one or more additional suppliers. An additional 30 were actually dispensed under generic name.

Among these, the priority for clinical trials was determined on the basis of the following criteria:

- The product is generally considered as a "critical" drug–that is, required for the control of a disease, rather than for the alleviation of temporary symptoms.
- It is generally dispensed in solid form–as a tablet or capsule.
- The active ingredient is relatively insoluble.
- Particular attention should be given to those drugs which had previously been the subject of reported or suspected nonequivalency or therapeutic failure.

A number of drugs meeting these criteria–together with a few others chosen for special study–were selected by the Task Force in consultation with representatives of clinical medicine, pharmacology, pharmacy, brand-name and generic-name manufacturers, the Food and Drug Administration, and other governmental agencies. Among these drugs, listed in alphabetical order, were the following:

Aminophylline	Para-amino-salicylate, sodium
Bishydroxycoumarin	Potassium penicillin G
Chloramphenicol	Potassium penicillin V
Chlortetracycline	Prednisone

Diethylstilbestrol	Quinidine
Diphenhydramine	Reserpine
Diphenylhydantoin	Secobarbital sodium
Erythromycin	Sulfisoxazole
Ferrous sulfate	Tetracycline
Griseofulvin	Thyroid
Hydrocortisone	Tripelennamine
Isoniazid	Warfarin sodium
Meperidine	
Meprobamate	
Oxytetracycline	

(It must be emphasized that inclusion in this list does not necessarily indicate that any or all generic-name products are or are not biologically equivalent.)

Biological equivalency studies on these products in human volunteers began late in 1967 in the FDA laboratories; at Georgetown University, under an FDA contract; and at the Public Health Service Hospital in San Francisco.

(Detailed results of these investigations are not presented in this report. Since they will obviously be of practical concern to physicians and scientists, the data are being announced–as quickly as they become available–in the usual medical and technical publications. It is expected that products will be removed from the market as an essential step in improving the quality of health care where legally and clinically significant nonequivalence has been established.)

As an important part of these trials, attempts are being made to determine whether any observed differences in biological availability could be correlated with differences in any physico-chemical characteristics of the product. Such physico-chemical differences could presumably be utilized in developing new and improved specifications for drug quality testing.

The Task Force recommends that the present clinical trials to determine the biological equivalency of important chemical

equivalents should be continued by the Department of Health, Education, and Welfare on a high priority basis.

In earlier interim reports, the Task Force indicated that these biological equivalency trials would be reasonably up-to-date by 1970.

As a more realistic projection, we find that the drug quality studies undertaken by the Food and Drug Administration are expected to be adequately if not completely up-to-date by 1971, and thus will provide reasonable assurance of uniform drug quality by that time.

Drug Cost and Clinical Equivalency

Various proposals have been presented under which the Secretary of Health, Education, and Welfare, in Medicare and other drug programs, would be empowered to provide reimbursement at a higher price if the manufacturer could substantiate a claim that his product possessed "distinct therapeutic advantages" over a chemical equivalent product. These suggestions have been carefully considered by the Task Force.

Although this double-standard approach appears to present certain economic advantages, it also presents obvious clinical hazards.

In the case of chemical equivalents available from two or more sources, we are convinced that the primary objective should be to provide the physician with every reasonable assurance that all chemical equivalents of the same drug on the market–when administered in the same manner and in the same dose–will give essentially equivalent clinical results. Unless the drugs perform reliably in the clinical situation, the physician will find himself in an intolerable situation, with the possibility that he may be placing the health or even the life of his patient in jeopardy.

Accordingly, when the patent on a product expires and it becomes possible to market chemical equivalents, the original drug product–by virtue of the clinical experience accumulated through its use, and because physicians will have become familiar with its characteristics–should serve as the *reference product*.

As recommended by the Food and Drug Administration, any generic-name counterpart thereafter proposed for introduction should be required either (a) to match the reference product, through conformity with all pertinent USP, NF, or other compendium standards, and, when required by the Secretary, presentation of appropriate test data to demonstrate essentially equivalent biological availability, or (b) to present acceptable clinical evidence of safety and efficacy through the New Drug Application procedure.

A chemical equivalent which does not meet one or the other of these requirements should not be accepted for Federal reimbursement or purchase, and should not be approved for shipment in interstate commerce.

> ***We therefore find that there should be uniform standards of quality and efficacy for each drug in any Federally-supported drug program, and that it would be inappropriate to provide for differential cost ranges for products sold under brand or generic names.***

Drug Standards

In the United States, the two most important official compendia of drug standards and specifications are the U.S. Pharmacopeia (USP) and the National Formulary (NF). Both have long and distinguished histories, and are highly regarded by physicians and scientists.

Although both publications have clearly stated that they cannot guarantee it, their standards and specifications have been widely presumed to assure the clinical equivalency of chemical equivalents.

The recent finding that some chemical equivalents are not biologically equivalent, even though they conform to existing USP and NF standards, has shown that certain of these standards may require revision.

During the past year, representatives of both USP and NF have been cooperating closely with the Task Force to meet this challenge. It is expected that existing specifications will be tightened where indicated and possible, and that these modifications will be incorporated in the revised USP and NF editions now in preparation.

The Task Force commends the U.S. Pharmacopeia and the National Formulary for their prompt and responsible approach to the problem of clinical equivalency.

Quality Control

The establishment and enforcement of product standards and specifications represents one important approach to the problem of drug quality and clinical equivalency.

Another is the establishment and rigid enforcement of appropriate quality control standards in all aspects of drug production and packaging. The Task Force has already recommended that a registration and licensing system be considered under which drug producers and packagers would be required to conform to a code of Good Manufacturing Practices and other criteria.

> ***We likewise recommend that adequate financial support should be provided to the Food and Drug Administration for necessary educational and inspection operations so that acceptable quality control methods can be instituted and properly maintained in all drug manufacturing and packaging establishments.***

> ***We recommend that the Food and Drug Administration should be authorized to provide additional support, including grants-in-aid, to State and local agencies in order to improve quality control of prescription drugs in intrastate commerce.***

The enforcement of an acceptable quality control program may be expected to have these effects:

- Many reputable manufacturers, both large and small, already maintain acceptable quality control programs, and will merely be obliged to continue them.
- Some manufacturers may elect not to institute such programs, and their products would therefore be found unacceptable for shipment in interstate commerce.
- Other manufacturers will elect to institute and maintain acceptable quality control methods. This may result in slightly higher production costs, which the manufacturers would most probably cover by setting slightly higher prices on their products.

The Task Force is strongly convinced that the added investment of Federal funds to require acceptable quality control methods, and the slightly higher drug prices that may result in some instances, would be more than justified by the improvement in drug quality that would be achieved.

We have given careful consideration to proposals for the placement of fulltime Food and Drug Administration inspectors in every drug manufacturing plant–large and small–but believe this would involve unjustifiably heavy expenses and inappropriate use of skilled manpower.

We have also considered proposals for the extension of batch certification–now applied mainly for insulin, antibiotics and biologicals–to all drugs, requiring FDA testing and approval at the manufacturer's expense before any batch may be released for distribution. We feel this would place an unnecessarily heavy and costly burden on manufacturers which would be reflected in unnecessarily higher prices to consumers.

Instead, we believe that further study is needed on the use of self-certification, with each manufacturer instituting and maintaining a quality certifying program approved by FDA.

CHAPTER 7
GENERIC PRESCRIBING AND DRUG COSTS

In recent years, as noted elsewhere, the possibility of reducing prescription drug costs by inducing or requiring the prescription of low-cost chemical equivalent products wherever available–an approach known as generic prescribing–has evoked some interest.

Savings can obviously be made by such a method. For example, it has been testified that some patients are required to purchase Meticorten, at $8.50 for 30 tablets, when the drug is available under its generic name of prednisone at $2.58 for the same number of tablets. Similarly, they pay $7.06 for 100 tablets of Serpasil, although it is available under the generic name of reserpine at $2.91. They purchase Achromycin at $5.56 for 16 capsules, even though it is available under its generic name of tetracycline for $3.83.

The substantial savings which could be made by generic prescribing in such specific cases are apparent. The significance of such differences when measured against a total drug program, however, has not heretofore been examined. Establishment of the Master Drug List in this Task Force study has afforded an opportunity to examine the situation in more detail.

Among the 409 products in the MDL were 86 which were dispensed under brand name, but which were no longer protected by patent and could have been purchased under a generic name from one or more additional suppliers. In the case of 23 of these multiple-source products, however, the chemical equivalents were available at only the same or higher cost, and offered no opportunities for savings.

There remain, therefore, 63 products which could have been obtained from multiple suppliers at a cost distinctly lower than that of the brand-name product actually dispensed.

For these 63 products, the use of low-cost chemical equivalents could have reduced the total acquisition cost to the retailer from nearly $74.9 million to $33.4 million, representing a potential saving of $41.5 million, or 55.3 percent at the wholesale level.

The saving to consumers would depend in part on the markup established by the pharmacist:

- If the markup were set so the pharmacist would receive the same gross profit as before ($1.81 per prescription)–neither gaining nor losing by dispensing a low-cost chemical equivalent–the total retail price would be reduced from $150.0 million to $108.5 million. This would represent a saving to consumers of the full $41.5 million, or 27.7 percent on the 63 drug products involved.
- If the markup were set at $1.50 per prescription, the saving would be $54.4 million, or 36.3 percent.
- If it were set at $2.00 per prescription, the saving would be $33.8 million, or 22.5 percent.

The impact of such potential savings on the entire drug program would be less significant. Thus, when measured against the total retail cost of $612.3 million for all 409 drugs on the Master Drug List, a saving of $41.5 million would have these effects:

- A saving of 8.0 percent with a $1.50 markup by the pharmacist.
- A saving of 6.1 percent with a $1.81 markup (which was the actual markup received by the pharmacist on these prescriptions).
- A saving of 5.0 percent with a $2.00 markup.

It must be emphasized that these calculations are based simply on cost levels for these drug products as they existed in 1966. They are not concerned with any differences which might have existed in the quality of the respective products, nor with any administrative or other costs which would be involved in any drug program requiring generic prescribing, nor with any use of formularies or other guidelines.

Savings might be more substantial in later years, since patent protection would expire on some drugs listed as single-source products on the 1966 Master Drug List, and low-cost generic could appear as competitive items. On the other hand, it appears reasonable to expect that new patented drugs would be added year after year to the list of most frequently used products, and the overall change would therefore not be appreciable.

Although the savings indicated above as a percentage of a total program–about 5 to 8 percent–may not seem large, any economy of the order of $41.5 million per year can scarcely be considered insignificant. Moreover, such savings would involve many products used in long-term maintenance therapy, and thus would provide particular help to patients with chronic illness whose drug needs are often the most burdensome.

For example, among the 63 products for which low-cost generic-name counterparts were available, sizeable savings could be achieved notably with drugs prescribed for long-term use in the treatment of heart disease, high blood pressure, kidney disease, arthritis and related conditions, and mental and nervous conditions.

> ***The Task Force finds, therefore, that the use of low-cost chemical equivalents can yield important savings, especially in the case of patients with cardiovascular disease, kidney disease, arthritis, and mental and nervous conditions, and the use of such products should be encouraged wherever this is consistent with high-quality health care.***

CHAPTER 8
FORMULARIES

Another point of major controversy in recent years has been the use of a formulary in any proposed drug program. One of the obvious characteristics of this dispute is the lack of agreement on what kind of formulary the disputants are proposing or opposing. Thus, a formulary is apparently considered to be any one of the following:

- A list of *standard* drugs (as established by an officially designed body).
- A list of *recommended* drugs (as established by an individual, a group of experts, a medical society, a government agency, a hospital, an insurance plan, or a group of advertisers).
- A list of *approved* drugs (as established by a government agency, a hospital, or an insurance plan).

In this report, the word formulary is used to indicate a list of approved drugs or drug products–a drug listing restricted in order to achieve more rational prescribing, or economy, or both.

With the aid of expert consultants, the Task Force has reviewed a wide variety of such formularies, giving primary attention to those used by hospitals, and by American and foreign drug programs.

Foreign Drug Programs

A survey of national drug programs in a number of foreign countries has shown that formulary use ranges from restricted formularies, including only a few hundred items, to comprehensive formularies containing almost every drug on the market.

Some specify the drugs for which reimbursement will be provided. Others list the diseases for which drug therapy is covered.

Where formularies are employed, they are used to improve the quality of treatment as well as to control costs. They include only drugs which are believed to be safe and effective. In the case of the more restrictive formularies, those products which are considered by the medical community to be duplicative–offering no significant therapeutic advantages over other products on the market–are not listed. Where low-cost chemical equivalents are available, they are usually included rather than their more expensive brand-name counterparts.

There are usually provisions for reimbursement for an unlisted drug if the physician indicates that it is essential for the appropriate treatment of a specific patient.

In order to control rising drug expenses, there are moves in those countries which do not use formularies to require them in the future, and in those countries with large formularies to make these more restrictive.

Even in those countries with relatively restrictive formularies, but with the selection of drugs made by expert committees of clinicians and scientists, the utilization of formularies appears to be associated with general acceptance by practicing physicians and pharmacists, more intensive competition among manufacturers, relatively effective price control, and few, if any, reported problems related to therapeutic equivalency.

It is noteworthy that many major American drug manufacturers are able to compete successfully under such conditions, and have their products accepted for formulary inclusion.

Federal Programs

Under current programs, formularies are used in all military, Veterans Administration, and Public Health Service hospitals and clinics, but generally not in the drug vendor programs of these agencies. Each Neighborhood Health Center operating under the Office of Economic Opportunity may determine for itself whether it will use a formulary. As noted below, inhospital care under Medicare requires the use of an official compendium or a hospital formulary.

State Programs

Of the States with Medicaid or other welfare drug programs, thirteen are currently using a formulary system. These vary in the number of items from approximately 100 in Kentucky to almost 2,400 in Pennsylvania. Some States list specific drugs, while others list the diseases for which drug therapy is covered.

Most State formularies show classes or types of drugs that are not reimbursable, such as over-the-counter items, nonnarcotic analgesics, multivitamins, anti-obesity drugs, sustained release medications, and tranquilizers. Many place limits on maximum quantities, the number of permitted refills, or the maximum price for any prescription.

Some States encourage generic prescribing by basing reimbursement costs on the price of generic-name drugs.

There are usually provisions which permit reimbursement for an unlisted drug required for unusual situations.

In most instances, the State formulary was developed on the basis of recommendations by expert committees of physicians and pharmacists, although one State has used a formulary which is essentially a list of the most widely advertised brand name drugs.

Opinions on the advantages and disadvantages of such State formularies are divided. In some States, the use of a formulary is believed to be responsible for controlling costs, while in others a proposed formulary was rejected as impractical. In some, the use of a formulary has apparently been found generally acceptable by physicians, while in others it was opposed as implying that the State condoned second-rate medicine for welfare patients. Some State officials have held that a formulary, by restricting the choice of drugs, violated the rights of both physicians and patients.

Some physicians have voiced strenuous opposition to the use of a

State formulary developed by an expert committee, even while agreeing to practice in a hospital in which a similar formulary was developed by a similar group of experts.

The concept of formularies for State programs has not received any significant support from major drug manufacturers.

Although exact comparisons are impossible, it appears that average prescription prices in welfare programs are roughly 10 percent lower in those States using formularies. Although program costs can be limited by reducing the number of reimbursable items in a formulary, this is not necessarily so; for example, an overly-restrictive formulary may serve as an incentive to abuses which will raise total costs to very high levels. Similarly, even under an almost unlimited formulary, costs can be effectively controlled by limitations on maximum quantities dispensed and the number of permitted refills.

Private Insurance Programs

As in the case of State welfare programs, there is no agreement on the need for formularies in drug programs operated by unions, group practice organizations, insurance companies, and other private groups.

Where formularies have been applied–and applied most effectively–in such operations, their use has usually been associated with drug procurement on the basis of competitive bids.

Hospitals

Many American hospitals–including most of the major university and medical center hospitals–have developed formularies for their own use, partly as an educational guide to their staff physicians, and partly to cope with the inventory problems of their pharmacies.

The importance of such formularies was heightened by the Social Security Amendments of 1965, which stipulated that reimbursement for drugs used in the treatment of hospitalized patients in the Medicare program would be approved only if such drugs were included in the U.S. Pharmacopeia, the National Formulary, or similar standard compendia, or if they were in a formulary adopted in an accredited hospital by action of its pharmacy and therapeutics committee.

Enactment of the Federal Medicare legislation was followed in December 1965 by a resolution of the Joint Commission on Accreditation of Hospitals of the American Hospital Association and the American Society of Hospital Pharmacists to add pharmacy and therapeutics committee practices to the functions of an accredited hospital.

The American Hospital Association, the American Society of Hospital Pharmacists, the American Medical Association, and the American Pharmaceutical Association have joined in recommending a hospital formulary system for all hospital staffs "in the interest of better patient care."

Most hospital formularies include from several hundred to more than a thousand items. One major New York hospital has reported that a formulary of less than 500 drug products will cover all but 1 percent of the drugs needed for both inpatient and outpatient care.

Provisions are usually included for furnishing unlisted products required for unusual conditions.

Many hospital formularies encourage or require the prescribing and dispensing of chemical equivalents wherever these are available.

In developing these formularies, most pharmacy and therapeutics committees have generally found it unnecessary to include the overwhelming majority of combination of duplicative drugs on the market. In the case of hospitals, formularies make possible substantial economic savings since each hospital usually purchases its drugs on bids, producing keen competition between manufacturers on the basis of quality and price.

> *In general, the Task Force finds, American physicians have found a formulary acceptable and practical, especially when it is designed by their clinical and scientific colleagues serving on expert committees, when quality is considered at least as important as price, when the formulary can be revised at appropriate intervals, and when there are provisions for prescribing unlisted drug products where special clinical conditions so demand.*
>
> *We find that the use of a formulary is not a mark of second-class medicine, but is, in fact, associated with the provision of the highest quality of medicine in the outstanding hospitals in the Nation.*
>
> *Although use of a formulary is not a guarantee of high quality medical care, rational prescribing, effective utilization review, and control of costs, we find that the achievement of these objectives in a drug program is difficult if not impossible with it.*

In the interests of achieving the highest quality of medical care, we recognize the necessity of placing the fewest possible restrictions on the traditional right of physicians to prescribe according to their best clinical judgment.

Therefore, it seems appropriate that consideration should be given to the reimbursement or purchase of unlisted drugs or drug products under emergency conditions or when a physician demonstrates to an appropriate formulary committee or local pharmacy and therapeutics committee that this is essential for the well-being of a specific patient.

CHAPTER 9
QUALITY AND COST STANDARDS

Since implementation of the Medicare and Medicaid programs, increasing public attention has been focused on the cost of prescription drugs, particularly where Federal and State expenditures are involved, and on the possibility of utilizing suitable quality and cost standards to improve these programs.

Among the factors that are obviously involved are these:

1. *Drug Prices.* Many brand-name products are available under their generic names at substantially lower prices (see Chapter 7). The Department of Health, Education, and Welfare encourages the dispensing of such low-cost chemical equivalents where they are available and where their use is consistent with high quality health care. Federally-aided State programs, however, are under no obligation to follow this policy.
2. *Retail Markup.* Many pharmacists use a percentage markup of drug acquisition cost as a basis for establishing the retail price of a prescribed product. Others have adopted a fixed dispensing fee system which allows the same dollar return to the vendor, regardless of product cost. The relative advantages and disadvantages of these systems are now a matter of some dispute (see Chapter 3).
3. *Formularies.* A number of State programs limit reimbursement to specific drugs listed in a formulary. There is little consistency among these formularies, however, and many include drugs which are felt by the formulary committees of other States to be unnecessary for rational therapy (see Chapter 8).

4. *Clinical Equivalency.* Considerable controversy has occurred in recent years concerning the comparative efficacy of brand-name drugs and lower-cost chemical equivalents. Recent evidence of biological nonequivalency among a few drugs has created doubts among physicians and their patients about the efficacy of low-cost chemical equivalents in general (see Chapter 6).

5. *Government Expenditures.* The funds involved in these governmental programs are substantial. For example, the Federal and State governments spent about $208 million for prescription drugs for welfare recipients alone in fiscal year 1968. As implementation of State Title XIX programs continues, drug expenditures for the medically indigent will increase.

Legislative Action

The Task Force has carefully examined these and other factors in considering whether the Federal Government can and should impose more effective controls upon costs of drugs supplied in the programs specified by the House and Senate legislation.

One Task Force study, for example, was undertaken in response to Section 405 of the Social Security Amendments of 1967 which states that:

> "(a) the Secretary of Health, Education, and Welfare is authorized and directed to study . . . quality and cost standards for drugs for which payments are made under the Social Security Act . . . "

After consideration of the question of whether the Federal Government can exercise more effective controls on the costs of drugs supplied in the Medicare, Medicaid, and Maternal and Child Health programs, we presented a preliminary report as follows:

"1. The drug quality control studies [undertaken by the Food and Drug Administration] are expected to be adequately if not completely up-to-date by 1970, and this will provide reasonable assurance of uniform drug quality by that time.

"2. Establishment of reasonable cost and charge ranges for drugs provided under the Medicare, Medicaid, and Maternal and Child Health programs is feasible, and would reduce the cost of drugs to the Federal and State governments without sacrifice of quality."

On the basis of these preliminary findings, the Task Force recommended legislation to permit establishment of reasonable cost and charge ranges–the limits of Federal participation in reimbursement–for drugs supplied to patients in the three programs noted above. Thereafter, the Department endorsed legislation introduced in both the House (H.R. 16616) and the Senate (S. 3323) to establish such cost and charge ranges.

H.R. 16616 and S. 3323 were identical except for the wording of a proposed Section 1122 (a)(1)(A) in S. 3323. Each bill would have required the Secretary to establish guidelines showing a "reasonable cost range" for drugs dispensed to patients under health programs supported with Federal funds. The Secretary would be required to exclude from the reasonable range those prices which varied significantly from the price of the drug when sold by its established–or generic–name. He would be empowered to recognize a differential price for a brand-name drug, however, if the manufacturer could substantiate a claim that his product possessed "distinct therapeutic advantages" over a generic-name product.

Defined in each of the bills was a "reasonable charge" for drugs. This charge would be the lesser of (1) the cost of the drug within the "reasonable cost range" plus a reasonable fee or billing allowance, or (2) the pharmacist's "usual or customary charge."

In addition, the Senate version would have required the Secretary, in effect, to establish a formulary of drugs appropriate for use in the Federal and State programs–a feature that was currently under study by the Task Force and which, for that reason, was not endorsed by the Secretary.

In its study of these legislative proposals, the Task Force has been concerned with three major questions:

- Can the Federal Government provide adequate assurance that low-cost chemical equivalents will be of sufficiently high quality and provide essentially the same clinical effects as drugs sold by their brand names and often at higher cost?
- Is it feasible to limit Federal expenditures for drugs to those specified by the Secretary, with the expert advice of the medical community?
- Would the limitation of Federal expenditures for drugs to cost and charge ranges at which products are available by their generic names result in significant cost savings?

To all three questions, the Task Force has noted, the answer is yes.

Assurance of Clinical Equivalency

As noted above, we have found that the drug quality studies undertaken by the Food and Drug Administration are expected to be adequately if not completely up-to-date by 1971, and these–together with modification of existing drug standards, strengthened enforcement of the FDA's Good Manufacturing Practices regulations, and other steps–will provide reasonable assurance of uniform drug quality by that time.

Scope of Drug Benefits: Impact of a Formulary

The Task Force has examined the use of limited drug lists or formularies in hospitals and in a wide range of government and private drug programs in this country and abroad. In general, such formularies have been found to be useful guides to rational prescribing, and provide an effective means of cost control when developed by or in close cooperation with physicians who represent a broad spectrum of clinical and academic experience.

As a guide to predicting cost savings in Federally-supported drug programs, the experience of existing State formulary systems presents some difficulties. Each formulary may cover a different range of drugs, and many have restrictions on prescription quantities. Some limit the maximum price of an individual prescription or the total annual reimbursable expenses per beneficiary. Others restrict the use of particular drugs to certain disease conditions, some encourage or require the prescribing or dispensing of low-cost chemical equivalents, while still others are structured to favor brand-name drugs. Certain formularies omit "non-critical" drug classes, such as anti-obesity agents, nonnarcotic analgesics, antacids, or tranquilizers, and some include an "escape clause" which allows the dispensing of nonlisted drugs under certain conditions.

Although all of these factors may affect the costs of a drug benefit program to different degrees, it seems evident that the use of a restricted formulary can lower the costs of a drug program. This observation is borne out in reports on hospital formulary experience, a comparison of State welfare programs, and from the experience of social insurance programs in other countries.

> ***From a survey of the available evidence, the Task Force finds
> that the exclusion of certain combination products, duplicative***

drugs, and noncritical products from Federal reimbursement would contribute significantly to rational prescribing, and moreover, it seems reasonable to assume this could yield overall savings of at least 10 percent.

"Reasonable Cost" Ranges

If reasonable assurance of uniform drug quality is a logical prospect by 1971, the relative costs of chemically equivalent drugs will become a significant economic factor in drug benefit programs.

To analyze the potential cost savings which could be achieved by the dispensing of generic-name products, the Task Force initiated a study of the 409 drugs most frequently dispensed to the elderly. It found that 63 could have been obtained from a number of suppliers at a cost distinctly lower than the brand-name products actually dispensed. Maximum savings at the retail level would have ranged from 23 to 36 percent on these 63 drugs, or between 5 and 8 percent when applied to all 409 drugs.

From studies conducted by the Task Force and others, we find that establishing product cost ranges reflecting the cost of drugs generally available by their generic names would save approximately 5 percent at the retail level.

"Reasonable Charge" Ranges

Pharmacists usually apply the same pricing system to both drug and nondrug products by using a percentage markup, or margin, system. The markup for most items stocked in pharmacies averages about 50 percent of cost; for prescription drugs, it ranges from 65 to 100 percent or more of acquisition cost.

The American Pharmaceutical Association and other professional groups have advocated in recent years a flat dispensing fee to reflect actual professional costs. This approach is widely used among hospital pharmacies and some government and private drug insurance programs, and it is being adopted by a number of community pharmacies. Among the advantages cited for the fixed fee system are these:

- It removes an incentive to stock and dispense high-cost drug products when low-cost chemical equivalents are available.

- It makes clear that the dispensing function bears little relation to product cost and therefore emphasizes the professional service rendered by the pharmacist.
- By reducing the cost of high-price medications and increasing the cost of low-priced items, it eliminates the subsidization of some patients by others.

By itself, the employment of a dispensing fee reimbursement system does little to assure that reimbursement for pharmacy services will equitably achieve the desired economies. Rather, techniques should be developed so that the allowance will be designed to reflect only those expenses which are directly related to the dispensing function. No portion of program payments should be made for unrelated functions or for vendor services that are grossly inefficient.

Although the Task Force is convinced that significant program savings could be achieved through the application of techniques designed to improve the efficiency of vendor operations, it is impossible at this time to estimate the extent of these savings.

Administrative Procedures and Costs

The establishment of reasonable cost and charge ranges for drugs, as envisaged in S. 3323 and H.R. 16616, would entail new methodology and significant administrative costs. In addition to the drug quality and equivalency activities already under way, mechanisms would be needed at both the Federal and State levels to assume other new responsibilities involved in the proposed legislation. Among these would be the following:

1. Establishment of an expert advisory committee of physicians, pharmacologists, and pharmacists to advise the Secretary on the qualification of specific drugs and drug groups for cost reimbursement.
2. Improvement of Federal resources for the determination of drug acquisition costs, development of audit and compliance procedures, drug utilization review methods, and techniques to increase the efficiency of drug distribution.
3. Mechanisms to provide technical assistance to the States in developing and improving their drug benefit programs.

Although considerable experience has been gained at the Federal level–in part the result of Task Force activities–that would permit the swift and efficient discharge of some new responsibilities, others would take many months from the date of enactment.

We find that considerable time would be required to develop all the necessary administrative mechanisms. Therefore full implementation of such provisions as applied to Federal reimbursement for prescribed drugs cannot be assured in less than two years after enactment of appropriate legislation.

In a preliminary report to the Chairman of the Senate Finance Committee on an earlier similar proposal, S. 2299, former Secretary of Health, Education, and Welfare, John W. Gardner, submitted Task Force staff estimates of administrative costs which were in excess of $100 million during the first year and approximately $34 million annually after the first five years.

The bulk of this projected expenditure would have been for improved quality control and for drug product testing to be conducted by or for the Formulary Committee envisaged in S. 2299.

Secretary Gardner recognized, however, that the improvement of drug quality would benefit not only those eligible for drug benefits in Federally-assisted programs but all users of prescription drugs.

Indeed, since the staff report in 1967, the improvement of drug quality and the studies of clinical equivalency have become matters of high priority within the agencies charged with these responsibilities and these priorities are reflected in substantial budget increases.

Any necessary increases in Federal expenditures for the improvement of drug standards and quality control will have benefits which apply to all users of prescription drugs and should not be attached to the implementation of cost standards for drugs supplied in Federally-assisted programs.

Significant costs would be incurred, however, solely from the enactment of the proposed legislation. If the provisions of S. 3323 were to take effect in fiscal year 1972, we estimate that the net incremental costs to the Department of Health, Education, and Welfare and the State programs would be as follows:

	FY 1972 (millions)	Subsequent years (millions)
Determination of "appropriate" drugs	$ 1.3	$ 0.7
Determination of product costs	1.4	0.6
Determination of dispensing allowances	0.9	0.5
Publication of drug lists, guides, and other informational materials	1.2	1.2
Technical assistance to State agencies and compliance review (Titles V and XIX)	1.6	0.6
Incremental costs of State agency audit (Titles V and XIX)	0.4	0.4
Review of drug providers (for exemption from provisions of the act–Title XVIII)	0.5	0.3
Costs of administration to non-exempt providers (Title XVIII)	0.4	0.3
Total administrative costs	$ 7.7	$ 4.6

Projected Savings

At the present time, Medicaid programs are in effect in 43 States and other jurisdictions. Of these, 36 provide reimbursement for the costs of prescription drugs. Drug expenditures under the program totaled $239.5 million in fiscal year 1968, approximately 7.8 percent of all Medicaid expenditures. In addition, $3 million was spent for drugs under the various Maternal and Child Health programs. It is anticipated that joint expenditures for drugs under these programs may rise to approximately $300 million by mid-1971.

If drug expenditures do, in fact, reach $300 million in that year, and if the projected savings outlined earlier in this report are applied, the following program savings could be expected:

		Savings (Millions)
Potential savings		
Establishment of "reasonable cost ranges"	$ 15.0	
Specification of cost-reimbursable drugs	30.0	$ 45.0
Less administrative expenses (first year)		7.7
Net Savings (first year)		*$37.3*

These figures could vary substantially, however, with such factors as the development of an out-of-hospital drug benefit program under Title XVIII, the costs to drug producers of developing and supplying data needed to substantiate drug quality, the extent to which the States develop their own mechanisms for limiting drug expenditures, and the effectiveness with which Federal quality and cost standards are applied at the State level.

From a consideration of the projected costs and savings, we reaffirm our earlier finding that establishment of reasonable cost and charge ranges for drugs provided under the Medicare, Medicaid, and Maternal and Child Health programs is feasible, and would reduce the cost of drugs to the Federal and State governments without sacrifice of quality.

CHAPTER 10
DRUG CLASSIFICATION AND CODING

Within a few years, it may be expected that prescription drug benefits under existing public and private programs will involve several hundred million prescriptions annually.

Without a universal coding, classification and identification system—a common language for communicating essential information—the Task Force finds that the administrative and accounting costs for processing such a volume will inflate program costs beyond acceptable limits.

To find methods of coping with this problem, the Task Force appointed *ad hoc* committees of experts on classification and coding which began a series of meetings in July 1967. In these conferences, criteria were established for a system under which all known pharmaceutical preparations could be identified and desired data stored and retrieved by use of existing and planned electronic data processing techniques and equipment.

Classification

The proposed classification system is now in final draft. It is the result of the joint efforts of representatives of the American Medical Association, the U.S. Pharmacopeia, the National Formulary, the

American Society of Hospital Pharmacists, the Drug Information Association, the National Pharmaceutical Council, the Pharmaceutical Manufacturers Association, the Food and Drug Administration, the National Library of Medicine, and various universities and State agencies.

Based on the vital necessity to relate cost analysis and utilization studies to how and why drugs are being used, the classification scheme is designed to accommodate products by categories reflecting their intended therapeutic action. This version makes it possible to place drugs in multiple settings. Final data collection will survey these settings and provide cost breakdowns and other cost analyses according to actual drug usage.

Application of the classification will have obvious importance for economic administrative procedures. More significantly, it will play an important part in developing information needed for improving the quality of health care.

> ***The Task Force recommends that the Department of Health, Education, and Welfare, the Department of Defense, and the Veterans Administration should test the proposed drug classification system to determine the feasibility of its eventual use in all public and private drug programs.***

We commend those whose efforts made possible the development of the system.

Coding

In the different aspects of drug manufacturing, distribution, sales, use, utilization review, accounting, cost analysis, and other marketing or administrative procedures, many different kinds of information may be needed. Basic to all of them, however, is information which will identify (a) the manufacturer, (b) the product, dosage form and strength, and (c) the package size, and which also is in a form which can be transmitted, stored and retrieved through electronic data processing systems.

Logically, the identification number would be assigned for all drugs on the market, and for any new drug at the time the New Drug Application is approved.

The number should be part of the required labeling, and ideally could be used to identify each individual tablet or capsule by printing techniques which are already being used by some drug manufacturers.

In addition, the number should be utilized in the coding for a proposed international adverse drug reaction reporting system which is now under consideration.

As a result of Task Force studies, it appears that an appropriate code can be developed by the use of a nine-character identification system utilizing both letters and numbers. The first three numbers would identify the labeler of the product (in most cases the labeler would also be the manufacturer), the next four would identify the drug, dosage form and strength, and the last two would identify the package size.

It is believed that such an identifying system would be able to accommodate a virtually unlimited number of different drug products.

The Task Force recommends that–

a. an appropriate identifying code number should be made part of all drug labels, package inserts, catalogs and advertising.

b. An appropriate coding system should be developed and tested by government and industry for this purpose.

c. After consideration of the results of this test, appropriate legislation should be introduced to require coding of all drug products in interstate commerce.

We commend those whose efforts are making the development of a new coding system possible.

As part of its activities in the field, the Task Force also supported development of an experimental National Drug Code Directory, prepared in preliminary form by the Food and Drug Administration to serve as a directory of essentially all prescription and over-the-counter drugs.

We recommend that the drug code adopted by government and industry be utilized in the National Drug Code Directory.

CHAPTER 11
UTILIZATION REVIEW

In any drug program, utilization review is a dynamic process aimed first at rational prescribing and the consequent improvement of the quality of health care, and second at minimizing needless expenditures.

In many hospitals, staff committees of experts have long taken the responsibility of reviewing the records of their fellow physicians and offering such advice or taking such disciplinary action as they deemed necessary. During the past two years, utilization review programs have been instituted to improve the quality of medical care under the hospital program of Medicare. Similar reviews are used in several American and foreign drug programs to improve the quality of drug prescribing.

It should be the responsibility of a program administration to institute a drug utilization review, and provide the necessary data and whatever statistical analysis may be required.

But the implementation–the establishment and improvement of guidelines, the provision for acceptable deviations, the limitation of irrational prescribing, the prevention of fraudulent practices, and other professional judgments–should be mainly the responsibility of clinicians, pharmacologists, and pharmacists who are widely respected as objective, well-informed, and appreciative of the needs of both physicians and patients, and who would work with their colleagues at the State and local level.

> *We find there is an urgent need for further research to develop and test various approaches to effective utilization review–approaches which would be most acceptable to physicians, pharmacists, consumers and others, and which would obtain their effective support.*
>
> *We therefore recommend that the National Center for Health Services Research and Development, in cooperation with State and local medical groups, community pharmacies, hospitals, and consumer groups, should support pilot research projects on prescription drug utilization review methods.*

CHAPTER 12
DRUGS UNDER MEDICARE:
THE ISSUE OF COMPREHENSIVE COVERAGE

Since July 1, 1966, the Medicare program–Title XVIII of the Social Security Law–has provided coverage for almost all of the inpatient hospital expenses of the elderly and for a significant proportion of their expenses for physicians' and other medical services. As a result, out-of-hospital prescription drug expenses represent the largest single personal health expenditure that the elderly must meet almost entirely from their own resources.

In 1967, for example, prescription drugs accounted for about 20 percent of the personal private health expenditures of older people.

It is not surprising, therefore, that there has been much interest on the part of the Congress in covering out-of-hospital prescription drugs under Medicare. Since 1965, more than 50 bills have been introduced to cover drugs under this program. In 1966, a bill that would have covered prescription drugs under the Supplementary Medical Insurance Program (Part B of the Medicare program) was passed by the Senate, but the drug coverage provision was deleted in conference.

Similar interest on the part of the Executive Branch of the Federal Government was marked by the presidential directive that led to establishment of the Task Force on Prescription Drugs to study the problems involved in covering the cost of prescription drugs under Medicare. At the request of the Task Force, the Social Security Administration–the agency that would have primary responsibility for administering a drug benefit under Medicare–has taken main responsibility for studying the feasibility of alternative methods of covering out-of-hospital prescription drugs.

The primary reason for proposing that an out-of-hospital drug benefit be provided for the elderly under Medicare, rather than through some other means, is based on the fact that the Medicare program has proven to be a highly successful method of financing the high health costs incurred by the elderly. The program has gained widespread acceptance among the elderly themselves, the health care community, and those who contribute to the program. Coverage of out-of-hospital prescription drugs under Medicare would relieve the elderly of part of the economic burden associated with their high drug costs, and would also represent an important step in assuring that their total health care needs are adequately met. The Task Force believes that, to the extent that it is possible to do so without incurring unreasonably high administrative costs, an out-of-hospital drug program under Medicare should be designed in such a way that beneficiaries will be able to understand it easily, and will not be unduly burdened by the procedures for obtaining benefits.

The specific provisions of an out-of-hospital drug benefit under Medicare would have to be developed within the context of the administrative complexities involved in a drug benefit and the funds available for financing the new benefit. One of the most important considerations affecting these factors is the scope of the drug benefit to be provided.

Most of the legislative proposals for coverage of drugs under Medicare that have been introduced in the Congress thus far would have covered drugs on a comprehensive basis–that is, they would have covered the majority of the approximately 1200 different legend drugs on the market.

There is no doubt that such comprehensive coverage of drugs under Medicare would represent a considerable financial benefit for the elderly. Comprehensive coverage, it should be noted, does not imply coverage of all prescription drugs. Even the most nearly complete drug coverage provided in existing programs have limits on the drugs covered and establish limiting conditions under which payment for drugs would be made; for example, it is the common practice of many private insurance and other drug programs to exclude from coverage certain classes of drugs–e.g., anti-obesity drugs, multiple vitamins, nonnarcotic sedatives, antacids, etc.–whose medical necessity is often marginal. However, even after such drugs are excluded from coverage, the numerous and complex administrative problems and very high program costs that would be involved in covering the remaining drugs present strong arguments for not attempting to provide comprehensive coverage in the first stages of a new drug program under Medicare.

Administrative Problems

One very important consideration in developing a plan for the coverage of drug expenses of elderly people is that there would be an extremely large volume of bills for covered services if comprehensive coverage were provided.

- It is estimated that the elderly would obtain more than 300 million prescriptions in the first year of operation.
- These prescriptions would be obtained through some 54,000 community pharmacies and some 3,000 hospital outpatient departments, as well as other providers of drugs to outpatients (e.g., mail-order firms, extended care facilities, clinics, and dispensing physicians).

The magnitude of the administrative tasks implied by these figures can be appreciated by comparing them to operating statistics for the first year of Medicare:

- During fiscal year 1967, some 10.4 million claims were processed by the hospital insurance intermediaries, while 26.5 million claims were processed under the medical insurance part of the program–a total of less than 37 million claims.
- The covered services were provided by about 7,000 participating hospitals, 4,000 extended care facilities, 2,000 home health agencies, 2,000 independent laboratories, and more than 170,000 physicians.

Even though the pharmacists and other drug vendors submitted combined or composite bills for covered drugs, the volume of items to be processed under a comprehensive program would obviously be much greater than that under the present Medicare program. While the claims transactions with respect to prescription drugs would be fairly simple, and there would be no variation in the types of data required for each claim, preliminary administrative planning indicates that each prescription involved in a claim for drug benefits would entail a minimum of half a dozen items of information, all of them subject to being transcribed incorrectly, either by machine or by hand.

Under these conditions, it is clear that efficient administration of a drug program of such a magnitude requires a fully automated data processing system operating with a high degree of accuracy.

During the beginning stages of any major new program, the use of automated data processing systems frequently involves problems arising from faulty operation of newly installed equipment, improper programming and human error. Furthermore, in any automated process, some items need to be handled manually because they contain discrepancies. If anything approaching the percentage of items for manual handling usually considered acceptable were excepted from the automated drug claims process, there is a possibility that the claims process would suffer a serious breakdown.

While these problems generally diminish over time and as experience is gained, it seems quite essential at the beginning to limit the number of claims items to be processed to a size which would keep within acceptable limits the risks involved in establishing a new system of processing. And even under a limited drug coverage program, it would be desirable to provide for a considerable period of time to prepare for administration of the benefit.

An additional consideration is that a large proportion of prescriptions are relatively inexpensive. Under these circumstances, it is difficult but important to develop provisions for administration so that costs associated with claims processing would not be excessively high in proportion to the benefits received by the beneficiary.

A final consideration is that in terms of the scope of benefits that would be involved, there is only limited useful precedent in either private insurance or governmental drug programs from which to develop the administrative procedures needed if a comprehensive drug benefit of this magnitude were provided.

Cost of Comprehensive Coverage

Another important consideration relating to coverage of most of the prescription drug expenses of the elderly under Medicare is the high cost associated with such coverage. The Social Security Administration had indicated that the "high-cost" estimate for comprehensive coverage of prescription drugs under Medicare, assuming a 20 percent co-insurance and an effective date of 1971, would be $1.6 billion, exclusive of administrative costs. (This estimate assumes a per capita acquisition of 21.5 prescriptions, and an average price per acquisition of $4.58.)

The Case for Less-Than-Comprehensive Coverage

There are, then, sound reasons why, in the first stages of administering a drug program, the Medicare program should not attempt to meet virtually all of the drug expenses of all older people. In fact, there is some question whether it would ever be desirable to attempt to provide insurance protection against small annual drug expenditures. A more effective use of program funds might result if an effective system could be found for limiting the benefits in a way that would concentrate the protection where it is most clearly needed.

Adoption of a limited approach would be consistent with the purpose and philosophy underlying Medicare–and, in fact, the entire social security program. The program is designed to encourage beneficiaries to build additional protection through private insurance, individual savings, and private pension plans. And, while cash benefits are intended to provide meaningful wage replacement for fulltime regular workers, it has always been recognized that some individuals will have special needs that cannot be met through the combination of private initiative and the social insurance mechanism, and that there will be a continuing but declining need for assistance programs.

Similarly, the Medicare program, by providing protection against only those expenses which the elderly as a group have the greatest difficulty in meeting, assumes that individuals will continue to meet part of their own health expenses, that private health insurance will be of continuing importance in meeting the health care expenses of the elderly, and that medical assistance programs will play a continuing, though supplementary, role.

The Task Force finds that, because of the numerous and complex administrative problems and the high program costs involved in providing drug coverage under Medicare, it would be desirable–at least at the outset–to provide the benefit on a less-than-comprehensive basis.

CHAPTER 13
DRUGS UNDER MEDICARE:
COVERAGE UNDER PART A OR PART B

Under present law, the Medicare program consists of two separate parts, the hospital insurance program (Part A) and the supplementary medical insurance program (Part B).

- Under the hospital insurance program, which is financed through payroll contributions, virtually all of the elderly are entitled to benefits.
- In contrast, enrollment in the supplementary medical insurance program is voluntary, and medical insurance benefits are provided on a current-premium basis.

All of the proposals thus far introduced in the Congress to cover out-of-hospital drugs under Medicare would have provided this coverage under Part B of the Medicare program, and the Congress requested that the Secretary of Health, Education, and Welfare study the possibility of coverage under Part B; because of certain problems evident in covering prescription drugs under Part B, however, consideration has also been given to coverage under Part A.

In terms of the coverage of out-of-hospital drugs under Medicare, there are two fundamental aspects–eligibility for benefits and financing–in which coverage under Part B would have significantly different results from those under Part A.

While there are other important differences between the two parts of the Medicare program–especially in the areas of claims processing and reimbursement–these do not represent fundamental differences between the two programs, and could be modified if a drug benefit were added. For example, while under Part B at present the beneficiary generally initiates a claim for benefits, if a drug benefit were added to Part B it would be entirely feasible to rely on drug vendors to initiate the claim for drug benefits. (These nonbasic differences between Part A and Part B are discussed where appropriate in Chapters 15 and 16, which discuss issues relating to administration and reimbursement.)

Eligibility for Benefits

Participation in Part B depends at least in large part on an individual's ability to pay the monthly premiums, which are matched by contributions from Federal general revenues. As of July 1, 1968, 18.6 million people aged 65 or over–95 percent of the elderly–were enrolled under Part B of the Medicare program.

It is clear that most of the elderly feel they need the protection that Part B offers, and it is expected a high proportion of them will continue to participate in this voluntary part of the program. Nonetheless, while some of the elderly who have not enrolled under Part B either feel they do not need or do not want the protection offered by the program, it is likely that many who have not enrolled simply cannot afford the monthly premium. There is, of course, no way to predict what effect future increases in the Part B premium will have on enrollment under that plan.

If, on the other hand, out-of-hospital drugs were covered under Part A of Medicare, virtually all people now aged 65 or more would be automatically eligible for the new benefit. As of July 1, 1968, 19.7 million persons aged 65 or more–99 percent of the elderly–were eligible for hospital insurance under Medicare, including some 2 million individuals who were not insured for social security or railroad retirement cash benefits but who were eligible for hospital insurance under a special "transitional" provision, which is financed out of general revenues. (For men who attain age 65 after 1974-for women 1973-the special eligibility requirements provided under the transitional provision will merge with the regular requirements for social security benefits.) Individuals who are not eligible for benefits under the transitional provision include retired or active Federal employees and their spouses who are eligible for health insurance coverage under the Federal Employees Health Benefits Act of 1959 and who are not eligible for monthly cash benefits under social security or the railroad retirement program, and certain aliens who have been in this country for only a short time. It is expected that when the social security program is fully mature, from 95 to 98 percent of all the elderly will be eligible for hospital insurance benefits; ineligible persons will be only those who are not entitled to monthly cash benefits under social security or the railroad retirement program.

Another important consideration is that Part B eligibility lapses if the beneficiary elects to withdraw from the plan or if he fails to pay the monthly premium, while eligibility under Part A continues until a person's death. The experience of Title XIX drug programs indicates that the process of determining eligibility for benefits under a program in which continuing eligibility cannot be assumed constitutes one of the most expensive and troublesome parts of the claims process.

Financing the Drug Program

If a drug benefit were provided under Part B of Medicare, the program would be financed through the monthly premiums paid by beneficiaries, and the matching government contribution paid out of general revenues. This method of financing the drug benefit has several drawbacks.

For one thing, the additional premium needed to finance the benefit might prove sufficiently burdensome for the elderly who have to pay the present monthly premium so that more of them might decide to reject coverage under Part B. If a provision similar to Amendment No. 440 were enacted, providing for a drug benefit under Part B-which represents the approach introduced most frequently in the Congress-the cost of the benefit would be $4.60 per capita per month. (Under this approach, the beneficiary would be responsible for a $25 drug deductible in addition to the $50 Part B deductible under the present law, and payment would be made for 100 percent of the "allowable expenses" with respect to a given drug.) The monthly premium rate and the matching amount paid out of general revenues would each have to be increased by $2.30 to finance the new benefit. Amendment No. 440, of course, would have provided comprehensive coverage of drug expenses, and a more limited approach under Part B would be less costly.

It should be remembered, though, that in 1966, 53 percent of the Nation's aged individuals, and 11 percent of the families in which the head was aged 65 or over, had an income of less than $120 a month, while 29 percent of aged individuals, and 30 percent of families in which the head was aged 65 or over, had an income of between $120 and $240 a month.

Thus, many would find an increase in their monthly premium (currently $4)–even if it were less than $2.30 with a less-than-comprehensive coverage–to be a significant amount to pay from their low incomes. In addition, the insured person would also be responsible for the $50 annual deductible and a 20-percent co-insurance for covered medical services other than drugs, plus a $25 deductible applicable to covered drug expenses, and any amounts in excess of the "allowable drug expense" as well as any incurred health costs not covered under the Medicare program.

An additional consideration is that under Part B, increases in health costs or substantial increases in utilization of covered services must be paid for, through increases in the beneficiary's monthly premium, on a year-to-year basis as the cost increases occur.

In contrast, if a drug benefit were provided under Part A, the program would be financed through the regular contributory mechanism now used to finance hospital costs and the cash-benefit part of social security. Under this approach, an individual would pay for this protection during his working years, rather than at a time of life when he may well have low income, limited assets, and high health costs. In addition, increases in the health costs and the utilization of services covered under Part A can be assumed in establishing the contribution rates and thus averaged and paid for over a substantial period of time. Also, with contributions based on earnings, increases in the general earnings levels that can be expected to occur in the future will automatically provide additional income to the system to help meet increases in health costs.

The Task Force finds that while it would be feasible to provide coverage of out-of-hospital prescription drugs under either the hospital insurance (Part A) or medical insurance (Part B) programs of Medicare, there would be significant advantages, in terms of beneficiary eligibility and financing, in providing such coverage under the hospital insurance program.

CHAPTER 14
DRUGS UNDER MEDICARE:
ALTERNATIVE PROPOSALS FOR COVERAGE

Three possible methods of covering out-of-hospital prescription drugs under Medicare would appear to be of most value to beneficiaries with high drug costs, and would result in more limited program costs and a lower volume of claims than would occur under essentially full coverage. These alternatives are:

- Coverage of only those drugs important for the treatment of serious chronic illnesses which afflict the elderly.
- Coverage of most prescription drugs, combined with the use of a relatively large annual deductible applicable to drug expenses.
- Coverage of most prescription drugs, but with eligibility for the drug benefit restricted to social security beneficiaries who have attained age 70 or, alternatively, age 72.

These proposals embody, respectively, three common techniques for limiting the scope of a drug program: limiting the number of covered drugs; relying on a high cost-sharing factor; and limiting the number of eligible beneficiaries.

There are other techniques which would contribute to limiting program costs and which could be incorporated into any of the three proposals. Among them are these:

- Setting maximum limits on the cost of prescriptions to be reimbursed.
- Setting maximum limits on the quantity of a drug per single prescription for which reimbursement would be made.
- Discouraging over-utilization through the use of such cost-sharing mechanisms as co-payment or co-insurance applied to each prescription, and through utilization review.

These techniques are discussed in Chapter 16.

Coverage along the lines of any of the proposals discussed here could be provided under either Part A or Part B of the Medicare program.

Coverage of Long-Term Maintenance Drugs

Available data on drug use by the elderly support the hypothesis that coverage of only those drugs which are important for the treatment of chronic illness among the elderly, and which usually are required on a continuing or recurring basis, would concentrate the protection provided by a drug program where it is most clearly needed.

(As indicated in Chapter 1, there is wide variation among the elderly in the extent to which they use prescription drugs: those older people who have serious chronic illnesses use more drugs than those who are not chronically ill, and many of the drugs most frequently used by the elderly are associated with the serious chronic illnesses which afflict older people.)

Under such an approach, the Medicare law could provide that the Secretary of Health, Education, and Welfare would establish the list of specific drugs to be covered under the program. He would select those drugs which he finds are important in the treatment of the many serious chronic conditions which afflict the aged. Once a drug was so specified as a covered drug, reimbursement would be made without regard to the condition for which it was prescribed. The law might also include guidelines indicating how the list would be established. Also, to assist the Secretary in establishing the list of covered drugs, the law might provide for an Advisory Council on Drugs, including nongovernmental experts in pharmacology, pharmacy, geriatrics and other branches of clinical medicine, and representatives of consumer groups.

The statutory guidelines on the selection of drugs to be covered would authorize the Secretary to consider whether, both absolutely and in relation to other drugs in its therapeutic class, a drug was (1) of acceptable quality; (2) safe and efficacious, giving careful consideration to relative toxicity and taking into account studies by the Department of Health, Education, and Welfare, the Department of Defense, the Veterans Administration, and other agencies which the Secretary found to be appropriate; and (3) not unduly expensive in relation to its therapeutic efficacy.

The drugs selected could include, in addition to drugs which can only be dispensed upon prescription by physicians, certain drugs which can be dispensed without a prescription (e.g., insulin) but only if the Secretary found that such drugs were "lifesaving drugs," or that their withdrawal would be seriously harmful to individuals who had been using them, or that they provided acceptable substitutes in terms of economy and effectiveness for other drugs included in the list.

The guidelines would require that the list be reviewed and revised as neccssary, at least once each year, and that the Secretary be required to report to the Congress annually on the adequacy of the list and the cost of the drug benefits being paid.

If such an approach were adopted, it is estimated that the level cost of the new benefit, if provided under Part A of the Medicare program and assuming a $1 co-payment, would be 0.19 percent of taxable payroll (estimated on a "high-cost" basis and exclusive of administrative costs). On the assumption that 1971 would be the first year of operations, benefit payments in that year would amount to an estimated $720 million, with reimbursement made for about 135 million prescriptions.

A more limited approach might be the restriction of coverage to drugs which are important in the treatment of a limited number of specific, serious chronic conditions; for example, the list of covered drugs might be limited to those which are important in the treatment of cardiovascular disease, diabetes, kidney conditions and respiratory conditions. Such an approach would involve somewhat lower workloads and benefit costs than would be concerned in coverage of drugs important in the treatment of virtually all the chronic conditions of the elderly.

Coverage of such a limited number of drugs appears to be the most promising of the alternative methods of providing limited drug coverage that the Task Force has considered. This approach would have the administrative advantages of limiting the number of claims submitted for processing, and of providing the most protection to those of the elderly who, because they have recurring needs for drugs associated with chronic illness, can be assumed to have the greatest need for such benefits.

While such an approach might entail some problems of beneficiary understanding related to what drugs are covered, these problems do not appear to be insurmountable.

One indication of the feasibility of covering only a limited number of specific drugs for the treatment of chronic illness is that Norway and Denmark have adopted such a method of covering drugs under their social insurance health care systems.

In this country, a similar approach has been used successfully by the drug program of the United Mine Workers Welfare and Retirement Fund; in 1967 this program provided drugs for 500,000 eligible beneficiaries. (The closed panel United Mine Workers program is organized on a regional basis, with each region establishing its own formulary; the number of drugs in these formularies ranges from 64 to 148. Prescriptions are covered under the program only if they are obtained from physicians who have entered into participating agreements with the plan.)

Every effort would be made to help assure beneficiary understanding and to provide physicians and pharmacists with easily understandable information about the drug benefit, including an easy-to-use listing of all drugs covered under the program.

A more fundamental possible drawback to this approach is that there is a question whether widespread medical agreement can be reached on the drugs to be selected. Although it would, of course, be impracticable to compile a final list of "covered" drugs far in advance of the effective date of drug coverage, continuing work should be done to develop lists of drugs in the therapeutic categories associated with treatment of chronic illness.

One question that needs to be explored in depth is whether a medically acceptable list of important drugs used in the treatment of chronic illness would include a disproportionately large number of drugs that are often used in the treatment of *both* chronic and acute illnesses, and whether a significant portion of benefits might therefore go for prescriptions to treat acute, short-term illness.

As indicated earlier, data from the Master Drug List (which reflects some 88 percent of the prescriptions obtained from community pharmacies by the elderly in 1966) indicate that a relatively small number of drugs account for a high proportion of the prescription drugs used by these individuals. Although the Master Drug List provides merely an index of recent prescribing patterns, and does not necessarily reflect expert medical judgments as to what is good drug therapy or what drugs are most significant for treatment of serious illness, it serves at least as a guide to the number of frequently dispensed legend drugs in the various therapeutic categories associated with the continuing or recurrent treatment of the important chronic illness of the aged. The Master Drug List data indicate that there are fewer than 200 such drugs which are relatively frequently used for such purposes.

In order to achieve maximum benefits with whatever funds may be available, and to give maximum help to those of the elderly whose drug needs are the most burdensome, the Task Force finds that particular consideration should be given to providing coverage at the outset mainly for those prescription drugs which are most likely to be essential in the treatment of serious long-term illness.

Use of a High Annual Deductible

A second possible method of limiting the number of claims and program costs of a drug program under Medicare would be to pay benefits only where a beneficiary's drug expenses exceed a specified, relatively high annual amount.

Serious consideration has been given to a proposal under which virtually all legend drugs would be covered, subject to a $100 annual deductible, with a co-insurance of 20 percent to be paid by the beneficiary on drug expenses above that amount. Beneficiaries would be responsible for keeping records and submitting claims for reimbursement, and would be permitted to submit claims only after accumulating charges which equal the deductible amount.

Under this approach, the pharmacist would be asked to certify that a drug was available only on prescription and was provided for the use of the named beneficiary. The pharmacist's certification would appear on each receipt for a covered drug.

The beneficiary would collect and submit his receipts for covered drugs in a pre-addressed envelope furnished by the Social Security Administration. Reimbursement would be made directly to the beneficiary, on an indemnity or "reasonable charge" basis.

In comparison with comprehensive coverage, this proposal would result in substantial reductions in both program costs and claims levels. It is estimated that the cost of the proposal would be $405 million in the first year of operation, and that reimbursement would be made for about 100 million claims in that year. If the benefit were provided under Part A, it is estimated that the level-cost of the proposal would be 0.14 percent of taxable payroll (based on the "high-cost" estimate and exclusive of administrative costs).

Of the three methods of limiting the administrative burden of a drug benefit considered by the Task Force, this proposal could be designed in a way that would permit the highest degree of administrative simplicity. Not only would claims levels be greatly reduced, but a large part of the recordkeeping burden would rest with the beneficiary, rather than with the Social Security Administration. Moreover, the Administration would not, under some approaches, have to enter into agreements with the 54,000 community pharmacies or with the approximately 3,000 other dispensers of drugs. The process of negotiating such agreements and of maintaining ongoing relationships with participating drug vendors would obviously result in a substantial workload. An additional consideration is that drug vendors would not be required to keep records for reimbursement purposes.

Also, although this approach to coverage is patterned after the claims and reimbursement provisions in effect under Part B, there is no necessary relationship between the indemnity approach followed under Part B and the Part B financing mechanism. It would be possible, therefore, to follow the indemnity approach referred to above even if the eligibility and financing provisions of the new benefit were established under the hospital insurance part of the program.

The main drawback to an approach involving a $100 deductible is that, for a beneficiary with heavy drug expenses and limited resources, $100 is a very large amount of money, and a deductible of this size would mean that drug expenses would remain a real hardship to many beneficiaries. While a lower deductible amount could be established, this would result in increased workloads and program costs.

For example, a $75 annual deductible with a 20 percent co-insurance, provided under Part A, would involve benefit costs of about $535 million in the first year of operation, with reimbursement being made for an estimated 140 million prescriptions, and an estimated level-cost, exclusive of administrative expenses, of 0.18 percent of taxable payroll.

If the deductible were $50, assuming no other changes in the provisions just listed, benefit costs would be $710 million, reimbursement would be made for an estimated 190 million claims, and the level-cost would be 0.25 percent of taxable payroll.

Another drawback to a high deductible approach is the difficulty that beneficiaries would have in keeping track of their drug expenses. Under this approach, assuming an average cost of $4 per prescription, the beneficiary might have to accumulate as many as 26 prescriptions before he could be reimbursed for any of his drug expenses. Experience with the $50 annual deductible under Part B indicates that Medicare beneficiaries have great difficulty keeping track of their medical bills, especially those for small amounts, and supports the inference that the higher the deductible amount, the more serious the problems.

Furthermore, to a great extent the administrative and cost advantages of such an approach are based on the assumption that the administering agency would be engaging in only a minimum amount of claims administration. For example, since validity of a claim would rest primarily on a pharmacist's certification that the receipt was for payment of a prescription drug dispensed to given beneficiary, there would be opportunity for abuse of the benefit–such as beneficiaries procuring drugs for other members of their families or for their neighbors. The additional expenses involved in preventing such abuse would detract from the administrative and cost advantages of the proposal.

> *From a consideration of these factors, the Task Force finds that the use of an annual deductible to control costs presents opportunities that warrant further consideration.*

Pay Benefits at Age 70 or 72

A third approach to providing a limited drug benefit under Medicare which would reduce the cost and the number of claims involved would be to make the benefit available only to those who attain a certain age–for example, age 70 or age 72.

Under this approach, payment might be made for the great majority of the 1200 different legend drugs on the market, offering the benefits of a comprehensive program although to only a limited portion of the elderly. Only 65 percent of the present population aged 65 and over are 70 and over, and would therefore be eligible for benefits (53 percent would qualify if the eligibility age were 72).

If the eligibility age were set at 70 and virtually all prescription drugs were covered, the cost of the benefit–assuming a $1 co-payment–would be about $1.2 billion in the first year of operation, and the level cost of the benefit would be 0.42 percent of taxable payroll (estimated on a "high cost" basis). If the eligibility age were set at 72, benefit costs would be about $1 billion, and the level-cost would be 0.36 percent of taxable payroll.

Reimbursement would be made for about 240 million claims if the eligibility age were 70, and 205 million if the age were 72.

Costs and claims levels could, of course, be reduced further by means of cost-sharing provisions.

Apart from the problem of rationalizing age 70 or 72 as the age at which a particular Medicare benefit would become available when all other Medicare benefits are available at age 65, there is a question of whether such a new age limit would be the most effective means of concentrating protection where it is most needed. Medicare beneficiaries under age 70 or 72 who had very high drug costs might well have difficulty understanding a rationale which excluded them from coverage while paying for the drug expenses of people who, while older, were in somewhat better health.

Restricting benefits to those aged 70, 72 or more would reduce the size and cost of the program, but the Task Force finds that this is not a preferred approach at this time.

CHAPTER 15
DRUGS UNDER MEDICARE:
PROGRAM ADMINISTRATION

A number of important factors concerned with administrative policies and procedures have been considered by the Task Force. These include determination and demonstration of eligibility, the role of the drug vendors, the role of the administrative agency, certification by physicians, the question of utilization review, and the need for a delayed effective date.

Establishing Beneficiary Entitlement

If a drug benefit were included under Part A, a beneficiary's entitlement to the out-of-hospital maintenance drug benefit would be established at the same time as entitlement to hospital insurance benefits. In virtually all cases, such entitlement could be expected to continue until the beneficiary's death, and this fact would greatly simplify administration of the benefit. Once entitlement were established, the beneficiary identification procedures now used for the present hospital insurance program could be applied, and the pharmacist could assume that a beneficiary who presented an identification card indicating Part A entitlement was, in fact, entitled to Part A drug benefits. If the benefit were provided under Part B, such a presumption would be in error if the beneficiary had failed to pay his premiums or otherwise terminated his enrollment.

It is contemplated that an out-of-hospital drug benefit would be made available only to those beneficiaries who are not hospital inpatients. One consideration in so limiting eligibility is the fact that the great majority of inpatient beneficiaries are in participating hospitals and thus their hospital expenses, including the cost of drugs, are already being paid in large part by Medicare.

No payment for out-of-hospital drugs would be made where an individual was receiving drugs that were already being paid for by Medicare as part of his extended care benefits. For these individuals, out-of-hospital drug benefits would begin when their extended care benefits terminated. At the present time, many persons who receive extended care benefits under Medicare do not have their drug costs met as part of these benefits, since an extended care facility is not required to provide drugs. For these individuals, the out-of-hospital drug benefit would be payable under the new drug program, either to the beneficiary or to the drug vendor, depending on which reimbursement system was adopted.

Reliance on Drug Vendors

Administration of an out-of-hospital drug program would be greatly simplified if substantial reliance could be placed on community pharmacies and other vendors for initiating claims.

The major alternative would be a system under which the beneficiary paid for his prescription at the time of purchase, kept a record of his expenses for covered drugs, submitted claims for benefits, and was then reimbursed by the program on the basis of the covered expenses he incurred. With a population of beneficiaries that could be expected to undertake the recordkeeping involved in a considerable number of small claims, this procedure has much to recommend it. Under such conditions, it is probable that many small claims would not be filed, since the beneficiary would decide that it was not worth his while to file claims for very small amounts. The elimination of very small claims would not be altogether inequitable to the beneficiary, and would contribute to efficient administration. As noted above, reduction of claims volume could be achieved through the use of a sizeable deductible amount with respect to drugs.

This method of claims administration, however, might place an undue burden on many beneficiaries, which could be avoided if the claims process were initiated by the pharmacist rather than the beneficiary.

Administering the drug benefit through payments to drug vendors would have other important advantages in addition to relieving the claims burden that would be placed on the beneficiary if he were responsible for keeping records of his drug expenses. The vendor could submit claims at regular intervals on composite claims forms and receive periodic reimbursement for multiple claims. Recording of claims and collection of program data could be facilitated through such techniques as use of the National Drug Product Code. In addition, if only a limited number of drugs were covered under the program, primary reliance could be placed on the vendor to determine, by reference to the list of covered drugs, whether a particular drug would be a covered drug for which a valid claim could be submitted. Finally, use of automated data processing methods could be more readily employed where claims were submitted by the provider.

Reliance on the drug vendors in the claims and reimbursement process would also facilitate increased coordination of an out-of-hospital drug benefit under Medicare with the drug benefits available under other Government programs–principally Title XIX programs–which make payment directly to the drug vendor. In 1967, Federal vendor payments for out-of-hospital drugs amounted to $100 million and it is likely that all Federal programs involving vendor payments will be even larger in the future.

Reliance on vendors also would enable the Social Security Administration to take advantage of advances in electronic data processing capabilities, including equipment which would permit transmittal of claims information directly from drugstores to the agency processing the claims. At the present time, there are no proven communications systems for use in drugstores that would aid them in meeting the requirements of a drug program under Medicare by tying the drugstore into the automated data processing system. However, from the technological standpoint, there are no significant obstacles to the development of such systems once a program need has been established, and these devices could play an important part in efficient claims administration.

If substantial reliance were to be placed on drug vendors in the processing of drug benefit claims and in reimbursement, it is contemplated that vendors, like the providers of services under the present Medicare law, would be able to participate in the program only if they entered into an agreement to do so with the Secretary of Health, Education, and Welfare.

They would have to agree–

- To accept certain limits on the amounts they would charge program beneficiaries (these limits are discussed in Chapter 16).
- To submit bills with such frequency and in such form as may be specified.
- To make available drug and prescription records for drug audits.
- To keep such checks on the accuracy of the dispensing of prescriptions as may be provided under regulations.
- To meet such other conditions of health and safety as may be provided in regulations.

As drug vendors under the program, it would seem feasible to include community, mail-order and hospital outpatient pharmacies, clinics, and, in certain cases, dispensing physicians. In addition, extended care facilities participating under Medicare would be able to act as drug vendors under the program if they so desired. Where an extended care facility did not want to act as a drug vendor, as discussed above, covered drugs could be obtained from other dispensers of drugs, either by the beneficiary or on his behalf. It should be noted that some minor changes in the definition of the reasonable cost of extended care benefits would be required, to avoid anomalous situations which might arise because of the use of two different methods of making reimbursement for drugs. Some changes in regulations might be needed to assure that the Social Security Administration would not be paying more for a drug purchased from a retail pharmacist but furnished as an extended care benefit than the amount determined to be the "reasonable drug charge" (see Chapter 16) for that same drug furnished under a new drug benefit program.

It would seem desirable that physicians be permitted to act as drug vendors in the program only under certain conditions established by the Secretary. In determining reimbursement of such a dispensing physician, consideration should be given among other factors to the extent of any other professional services he performed at the time he dispensed the drug, and of any charges he made for those services; that is, the physician should not be reimbursed both for a dispensing charge as part of his "reasonable charges" as defined in the present Medicare law for professional services and also for a dispensing allowance in his capacity as a drug vendor.

The Task Force finds that it would be preferable for the vendor rather than the beneficiary to have major responsibility for keeping needed records and initiating claims, and to be reimbursed by the program.

Role of the Administering Agency

If a new drug benefit is added to the Medicare program, administrative responsibility should rest with the Secretary of Health, Education, and Welfare, with a primary delegation of authority to the Social Security Administration.

As the legislative specifications develop for the new drug program, and as the many complex problems of designing the most feasible method of administering the new benefit are resolved, it may prove to be desirable to enlist the assistance of nongovernmental organizations. The possible use of other organizations and their specific functions, however, will depend to a large extent on the resolution of other important administrative questions. For example, the nature of the automated data processing system that would be used in administering the new benefit would have an important bearing on the delegation of functions to outside organizations.

A highly sophisticated automated data processing system could function most effectively if the drug benefit were administered at the Federal level, but with appropriate consideration of the system's compatibility with systems used by other organizations. An additional consideration here would be the experience and proficiency developed by various organizations in administering drug-benefit claims by the time drug coverage is added to the Medicare program.

Because of the large number of claims which would be involved, the Task Force finds that a suitable automated data processing system could play a vital role in claims processing and other administrative activities, and should be developed and adequately tested.

Certification by Physician

The Medicare law excludes from coverage all services and supplies that are not medically necessary. This exclusion should apply to out-of-hospital drugs if they were covered under Medicare.

Under the present law, one of the primary methods of assuring that the Medicare program pays only for services which are medically necessary is the requirement that a physician certify to the need for the services received. In applying such a requirement to an out-of-hospital drug benefit, it is contemplated that the prescription filed with the drug dispenser would be the only certification required for most prescription drugs.

In the case of those drugs which are especially subject to abuse, coverage might be limited to instances in which the drug was prescribed for certain specified conditions. In such cases, the physician would have to provide information beyond the prescription itself.

Some form of certification–such as a physician's prescription–would also be needed with respect to any nonlegend drugs, such as insulin, which were included in the list of covered drugs.

Utilization Review

Utilization review is another technique for helping to limit payments to those for medically necessary services. The concept of utilization review is gaining widespread acceptance in the medical community as an appropriate means of discouraging unnecessary use of medical services and of encouraging improved patient care. By requiring as a condition for participation that hospitals and extended care facilities establish utilization review committees, the Medicare program has been responsible for the establishment of this machinery in most hospitals throughout the country. In the case of drugs, utilization review is being developed primarily to achieve rational prescribing.

It appears, however, that the problems involved in establishing effective utilization review procedures are probably greater for all out-of-hospital services than for services received inside an institution. In the case of drugs, the vast volume of prescriptions, the fact that a given prescription in itself provides information on only a small segment of an individual's total medical history, and the fact that there is not yet complete consensus among physicians on rational prescrib-ing–all these combine to present serious obstacles to the effective implementation of utilization review at the present time.

> ***The Task Force finds that to the extent that appropriate utilization review methods are developed, these should be applied in a Medicare drug program.***

The Task Force has already noted that there is a pressing need to encourage State and local medical societies and other concerned groups to work toward improving patterns of prescribing and has recommended strong support of research and experimentation with prescription drug utilization review methods.

Delay in Effective Date

In preparing this report, it has been assumed that the new drug program would become effective no earlier than two years after the date of legislative enactment. As discussed above, the relative administrative complexity of a drug program would depend on the details of design. Even the simplest form of administration would require a substantial tooling-up period.

CHAPTER 16
DRUGS UNDER MEDICARE:
PROGRAM REIMBURSEMENT

The specific provisions relating to reimbursement that are appropriate for a drug program would depend to a large extent on whether the claim is filed by the beneficiary or by the vendor of drugs.

For example, if the "high deductible" approach described above were adopted, with the beneficiary submitting his own claims, one feasible method of reimbursement would be the "reasonable charge" approach now used under Part B of the Medicare program. Since, however, most of the claims submitted would be for relatively small amounts, many claims would be filed a considerable period of time after the prescription was obtained, and the Social Security Administration would not have entered into any agreements with pharmacists on the records they keep, anything more than a very gross check on the "reasonableness" of the charges submitted by the beneficiary would be extremely costly and almost impossible to accomplish.

An alternative method would be to pay claims, once the deductible is met, on the basis of a schedule which would list a flat amount for each item paid for.

If, on the other hand, claims were to be submitted by the pharmacist and reimbursement were to be made directly to him, an entirely different approach to reimbursement would be possible. In evaluating the various possible approaches to such vendor reimbursement, emphasis has been placed on finding reimbursement techniques which would minimize disruptions in the pharmacist's customary methods of doing business–for example, techniques which would minimize the amount of additional recordkeeping and the amount of additional work involved in submitting claims, and which would allow the pharmacist to compute the program payment easily. Beneficiary understanding has also been stressed.

Other important considerations include the need for these factors:

- A reimbursement mechanism that would permit payment to be made on a current basis.
- A mechanism that would permit a reasonable check on the accuracy or appropriateness of payments made by the program without resulting in very high auditing and accounting costs.
- A method which would be acceptable to the drug vendor in terms of the total payment he receives, from both the program and the beneficiary.
- A method which would not reward inefficient operation, would not spend program funds for drugs that are not competitively priced in situations where competitively priced drugs are available, and would give the beneficiary an incentive to be conscious of comparative drug prices.

Guidelines in Law

It would seem desirable that guidelines with respect to reimbursement of providers of drugs would be stated in the law, but that the detailed reimbursement provisions would be established by the Secretary in regulations, after consultation with representatives of all affected groups.

This was substantially the procedure followed in establishing the principles of reimbursement for hospitals and extended care facilities under the present Medicare law.

The provision of a drug benefit under Medicare would, however, involve many more participating drug vendors than there are "providers of services" under the present Part A, and these vendors exhibit a considerable degree of variation in size, function, and volume of pharmacy business, as well as in methods of purchasing, maintaining inventories, and other methods of doing business. It would be important to the success of the program to give representatives of all classes of drug vendors the opportunity to present their views on reimbursement before the Secretary makes final decisions on this matter.

The guidelines in the law would state that reimbursement for out-of-hospital drugs would be made to qualified drug vendors on the basis of the "reasonable drug charge" for each drug, and that the "reasonable drug charge" would consist of cost elements relating to (a) the acquisition and (b) the dispensing of the drug, to be defined in regulations.

The guidelines in the law would also permit the Secretary, when establishing the reasonable charge, to take into account significant variations in the price at which the drug was made available to different classes of drug vendors with the result that the "reasonable drug charge" for a specific drug might vary among different classes of providers in different regions or localities. In addition, the guidelines would require that the regulations concerning the "reasonable drug charge" include a provision for periodic review in order to assure the continuing adequacy of the charge.

The Social Security Administration would carry on continuing studies designed to measure changes in the cost of the various elements included in the "reasonable drug charge."

Reimbursement for Product Costs

Determining the acquisition costs incurred by pharmacists and other drug vendors in furnishing covered drugs to Medicare beneficiaries is the aspect of vendor reimbursement on which probably the greatest amount of additional work is needed. Many different approaches have been utilized in various governmental and private programs in this country and abroad, but none has been demonstrated to be completely adequate. As the Task Force has noted elsewhere, extensive studies are needed on drug costs and drug prices, including further examination of the pricing structure of the drug industry, price changes among different categories of drugs, and related issues.

Among the methods considered by the Task Force as a basis of determining acquisition costs are these:

- Actual acquisition cost, as verified by audit,
- "Usual and customary" charges,

- Listed wholesale price,
- Fixed program payment.

Consideration has likewise been given to the significance of acquisition by generic name, government purchase, and establishment of price through government-industry negotiation.

Actual Acquisition Cost. Under the present Medicare law, providers of services are generally reimbursed on the basis of the audited actual costs of the covered services they furnish to Medicare beneficiaries. In the case of out-of-hospital prescription drugs, however, basing reimbursement on audited costs would involve substantial administrative expenses, and a significant degree of possible error. The acquisition cost of each covered drug furnished to a beneficiary would have to be determinable and verifiable through audit, yet it would be very difficult to determine with precision the cost incurred by the vendor in actually acquiring it.

Under the pricing system now prevalent in the drug industry, the published wholesale price of a drug product is subject to a complex system of frequently changing discounts, including discounts based on the purchase of other drug products, and cumulative discounts based on volume that may be computed after the end of the accounting year. Thus, in many cases the pharmacist's inventory may have been purchased at several different prices, and it is possible that the costs associated with determining the actual costs of acquiring drugs would be substantial.

"Usual and Customary" Charges. An alternative approach would be to base reimbursement on the pharmacist's "usual and customary" charges (including both acquisition and dispensing elements), thereby avoiding altogether any questions to the pharmacist about cost. In many cases, however, payment on the basis of customary charges would result in the program paying amounts for a drug that were far greater than the costs of the pharmacist in actually acquiring it. An additional problem is that a program of anything more than minimal checks on whether a charge was "usual and customary" would be exceedingly difficult to administer. Essentially, this approach to reimbursement would place no restraints on the prices that beneficiaries or the program paid for covered out-of-hospital prescription drugs.

While this would seem to be a feasible alternative if the beneficiary, rather than the pharmacist, were to submit the claims for drug benefits, it would seem to be the least desirable approach to vendor reimbursement, since it would offer no protection against unduly high prices to either the beneficiary or the program.

Listed Wholesale Price. Another alternative would be to base reimbursement on the listed wholesale price of a drug product, but, as noted above, these listed prices rarely have any realistic relationship with actual acquisition costs. The assumption here would be that any losses incurred by the program as a result of basing reimbursement on listed wholesale costs would be made up to the program in savings on auditing and other administrative costs.

It would seem desirable, if this approach were adopted, that *Red Book* and *Blue Book* prices not be relied upon as the sole determinants of the wholesale price of a given drug, but that price listings be compiled on a more current and reliable basis.

This approach would have the advantage of administrative simplicity. It would also permit the program to place some limits (discussed below) on the amounts paid by the beneficiary and by the program for a given drug.

Fixed Program Payment. Still another alternative would be to establish a fixed program payment with respect to each drug. Under this approach–comparable to indemnity fee schedules in many forms of health insurance–the program payment for a specific quantity of a drug product would be a single uniform amount, and would not depend on either the price paid by the beneficiary or the costs incurred by the pharmacist.

While this fixed payment would not have to bear any relationship to the costs incurred by the pharmacist, it *could* be based on an estimate of probable acquisition costs.

This approach would also have the merits of administrative simplicity and of being easy for the pharmacist to compute and for the beneficiary to understand. Here, too, it would be possible to impose certain limitations (discussed below) on the amounts paid by beneficiaries or by the program.

> ***The Task Force finds that reimbursement for product cost, as one element in the total cost of a prescription, may be considered on the basis of (a) "usual and customary" charges, (b) listed wholesale price, (c) actual acquisition cost as verified by audit, (d) a fixed program payment. Preference would be determined by the nature of the program.***

Acquisition by Generic Name

If the Medicare program and its contributors are to have the benefit of any reduction in costs which results from the availability of a drug from more than one supplier, and from the resultant price competition, it would seem necessary for the element of the "reasonable drug charge" related to acquisition costs to reflect the cost of acquiring the drug by its generic name, or, if lower, by its brand name. In most cases, this would be the cost of the drug when acquired by generic name.

It is recognized that under a program covering only a limited number of drugs, a requirement that reimbursement be based on the lowest cost of acquiring a given drug would result in some savings to the program. For example, data in the Master Drug List show that among the 82 drugs in the list that were prescribed for an average of 90 days or more per year, 11 were dispensed by their generic names and an additional 16 were dispensed under brand names but were available under generic name from more than one source. It is estimated that there could have been a 28 percent saving at the wholesale level if these 27 drugs had been purchased by their generic names at the lowest available cost.

If the number of covered drugs were not restricted, the potential saving from basing reimbursement on the cost of a drug acquired by generic name could be even greater. Thus, the Master Drug List shows that of the 409 drugs most frequently dispensed for the elderly in 1966, 30 were actually dispensed under their generic names, and an additional 86 products dispensed under brand names were drugs for which chemical equivalents were available. Together, these 116 drugs accounted for 39 percent of total MDL prescriptions, 37 percent of the MDL acquisition cost to retailers, and 32 percent of the MDL retail cost to patients. It is noteworthy that, in the case of 23 of the 86 drugs for which chemical equivalents were available, the chemical equivalents were available only at the same price as their brand-name counterparts, or at a higher price, and thus offered no opportunities for savings. Nonetheless, for the 63 multiple-source products which could have been obtained at a lower price if acquired by their generic name, the savings could have been considerable: the wholesale cost to the retailer of these products could have been reduced by about 55 percent. It should be noted that this hypothetical saving is based on the assumption that the lowest-priced generic drugs were all of acceptable quality and were available on a nationwide basis.

Although generic prescribing as a required approach presents many attractive features, it has certain evident drawbacks.

For example, any attempt to permit or require a vendor to dispense a low-cost chemical equivalent in place of a drug prescribed under its brand name would necessitate modification or repeal of the so-called "anti-substitution" laws now in effect in nearly all States.

There is nothing in these laws to prevent a physician from prescribing by generic name if he so desires. Similarly, there is nothing to prevent a physician from authorizing a pharmacist to fill the prescription with any suitable chemical equivalent. In a number of hospitals and drug programs, special prescription blanks are customarily used to provide such authorization routinely except when the physician specifies otherwise.

One drawback to basing reimbursement on acquisition of a drug by its generic name is that the Medicare beneficiary would have to bear the cost of the difference between the cost of acquisition by generic name and the cost of acquisition by brand name, in those situations in which the physician required dispensing by brand name.

This drawback, while serious, does not seem to be insurmountable. As noted above, even under existing laws, a physician may prescribe generically, or authorize the pharmacist to dispense an appropriate low-cost chemical equivalent. Every effort would be made to acquaint physicians with the names of the drugs covered under the program and with detailed information on how reimbursement would be made for covered drugs, as well as with information on the prices at which a covered drug was generally available.

Before a requirement was adopted basing reimbursement on the lowest acquisition cost, it would be necessary to provide assurance that all drugs on the market are of acceptable quality. In this connection, it should be noted that the drug quality control studies that were undertaken by the Task Force in cooperation with the Food and Drug Administration, the Public Health Service, representatives of the United States Pharmacopeia, the National Formulary and others are expected to be adequately up-to-date by 1971, and should provide reasonable assurance of uniform drug quality by that time. Further assurance could be gained by stipulating in the law that the Secretary could find that an out-of-hospital drug was a covered drug for reimbursement purposes only if it met the Secretary's standards as to quality.

Accordingly, the Task Force finds that reimbursement for product cost should be based on the cost of the least expensive chemical equivalent of acceptable quality generally available on the market.

At the same time, it is clear that the Department of Health, Education, and Welfare has the responsibility for keeping physicians, vendors, and the general public informed of the availability, quality and relative costs of chemical equivalents, and for urging physicians to prescribe low-cost chemical equivalents for all beneficiaries of Federal drug programs wherever this is consistent with high quality health care.

Government Purchase

Consideration has been given to other techniques which would prevent the Medicare program from paying excessively high prices for drugs, and one noteworthy technique–direct purchase of drugs by the government–was examined particularly by the Task Force.

The case for government purchase of drugs provided under Medicare is based mainly on two considerations: (a) the fact that if drugs were covered under Medicare on a comprehensive basis, the government programs (including Department of Defense, Veterans Administration and Public Health Service programs, as well as programs under the Social Security Act) would be paying, directly or indirectly, for a significant part–an estimated 46 percent–of the total domestic sales of the pharmaceutical industry by 1975; and (b) the assumption that if the government were either to purchase drugs directly, through competitive or negotiated bids, or to purchase patent and license rights and enter into contracts for producing drugs on the basis of the purchased licenses, the cost to the government would be much less than the cost of the same drugs acquired on a retail basis.

In the case of drugs still under patent, statutory authority already exists for the Federal Government to purchase such drugs from non-licensed manufacturers, either in this country or abroad, when this would be justified both by drug quality and by price savings.

In addition, the present drug procurement methods of several government agencies include plant inspection and analyses of quality of the drugs being purchased; if these procedures were adopted on a broad scale, along with purchase of patent or license rights, the government presumably could obtain a given drug at the lowest possible price without sacrificing quality.

There is, of course, widespread concern that prescription drug prices do not reflect price competition in the marketplace, and that as a result the price of prescription drugs is unduly high. The Task Force, however, does not recommend direct purchase of drugs by the government at this time as a means of controlling prices and conserving Medicare program funds. Direct government purchase of drugs for Medicare beneficiaries would have significant disadvantages. The primary purpose of the Medicare program is to provide, through the mechanism of social insurance, a method of financing the major health expenses of older people. Widescale direct purchase of drugs by the Medicare program would require that the program perform functions that are not usually thought of as social insurance, and would also introduce substantial alterations into the drug distribution system in this country.

> *Since the expressed purpose of the social security program is to provide assistance to beneficiaries, wherever possible, within the framework of the existing health care system, the Task Force finds that the direct purchase of drugs by the Federal Government for Medicare beneficiaries is not recommended at this time, but this approach deserves further study.*

A somewhat related approach would be establishment of acquisition cost on the basis of a price negotiated between the government and manufacturers–a method used in some national health programs. This approach presents some advantages, and warrants further study.

Reimbursement for Dispensing Costs

The reimbursement guidelines in the law would state that the elements in the "reasonable drug charge" which represent dispensing costs would include such factors as overhead costs associated with dispensing, a fair profit or return, extent of professional services provided, and other relevant factors.

The dispensing cost elements in the "reasonable drug charge" might take account of whether the drug product was a legend drug or an "over-the-counter" drug. In establishing the dispensing cost elements, the Secretary might also take into account substantial differences in dispensing costs associated with different classes of vendors in different geographical locations; in the interests of administrative simplicity, however, only a small number of classes of vendors would be established. The dispensing cost elements would be uniform for all vendors within each such class.

A number of approaches have been considered as the basis for determining reimbursement for dispensing cost. These include the following:

- A percentage markup based on the actual or estimated acquisition cost of the product.
- A fixed dispensing fee set to cover usual dispensing expenses plus reasonable profit and not related to the acquisition cost of the product.

Utilization of either approach presupposes that (a) the vendor is, in fact, aware of the actual acquisition cost of each drug, and (b) he is aware of his actual operating expenses involved in drug dispensing.

Percentage Markup

As described in more detail above, many vendors have traditionally established their dispensing compensation as a percentage–usually 65 to 100 percent or more–of the acquisition cost of a prescription drug product. It is based on the philosophy that the marketing of prescription drugs is, in general, not significantly different from the marketing of any other commodity.

Although it has certain disadvantages, application of the percentage markup approach has been found acceptable in many governmental and private drug programs.

Fixed Dispensing Fee

Based on the concept that dispensing services represent a professional function generally unrelated to the acquisition cost of a drug, some vendors have charged a fixed dispensing fee per prescription. This method now marks a number of State and Federal drug programs, including the CHAMPUS program for military dependents maintained by the Department of Defense. In the latter, for example, fees are set unilaterally by the government on a State-by-State basis and revised periodically as necessary to reflect changes in the costs of conducting business and to minimize any significant inequities.

If such a procedure were to be utilized for an out-of-hospital program under Medicare, it is presumed that the Secretary would take

into account such State or local differences, as well as differences in
the business expenses of different categories of vendor establishments.

> ***The Task Force finds that the preferred method of reimbursing
> dispensing costs would depend on the nature of the program. If
> the program provides for a specific dispensing allowance to be
> paid to the drug vendor, rather than payment to the beneficiary,
> either a percentage markup or a fixed dispensing fee would be
> feasible, with a fixed fee approach being preferable.***

Cost-Sharing Provisions

If reimbursement were to be made directly to the vendor, the most
feasible method of sharing the cost of the benefit with the beneficiary
would be for the beneficiary to be responsible for paying part of the
cost of each prescription.

Many drug programs, private and governmental, in this country and
abroad, have utilized such methods as co-payment, co-insurance, and
restrictions on reimbursable prescription costs or prescription quantities.

In some programs, for example, the beneficiary is required to
provide a co-payment of $1.00 or other specified amount for each
prescription. In others, he is required to pay 20, 25 or other percentage
as co-insurance. In a number of programs, restrictions are placed on
the total dollar amount of any prescription for which reimbursement
will be provided without special administrative approval, or on the
number of days' supply of any single prescribed drug.

Although complete data are not available, there are indications from the
experience of the programs in Great Britain and in North Carolina that use
of co-payment reduces the number of claims and the cost of a program.
Similarly, experience with the Medicaid program in Pennsylvania has
indicated that use of limitations or maximum prescription prices or
maximum quantities is associated with control of costs.

In terms of administrative simplicity and conservation of program
funds, a fairly high co-payment amount–in contrast, for example, to a
percentage co-insurance payment–would seem to be the most
advantageous approach, since it would eliminate a substantial number
of small claims. (Depending on the cost considerations involved in a
given program, refill prescriptions could be subject either to the same
flat co-payment as original prescriptions, or to a reduced co-payment
amount.) Consideration might be given to placing the co-payment
amount on a dynamic basis after the drug benefit had been in effect for

several years. (That is, the co-payment amount would be adjusted annually to reflect changes in the average per capita cost of drugs covered under the program.)

> ***The Task Force finds that any drug insurance program instituted under Medicare should include cost-sharing provisions, such as co-payment or co-insurance.***

> ***The Task Force also finds that consideration should be given to the use of restrictions on maximum prescription quantities or on maximum prescription prices as additional cost-sharing approaches.***

Limit on Amounts Paid by Beneficiaries

While it would seem to be important for an out-of-hospital drug benefit under Medicare to place reasonable limits on the amounts that beneficiaries pay for covered drugs, preliminary consideration suggests that it may not be feasible to require that the vendor agree that the program payment for a covered drug (plus any cost-sharing amounts) would represent full payment for that drug, as is the case with respect to Part A benefits under the present program.

One important consideration is the extreme difficulty which would be involved in arriving at an audited cost with respect to each pharmacy on which to base full-cost reimbursement. Another important factor is that not all overhead costs incurred by some pharmacists may be taken into account in the "reasonable drug charge"–an example of a cost element that may well be excluded is the cost of home delivery of prescription drugs. An additional factor is that if the program payment is based on acquisition of a drug by its generic name, but the pharmacist does not purchase by generic name, he will be incurring costs which the program would not meet. Given these considerations, it would seem necessary to permit the pharmacist to charge the program and the beneficiary together up to the amount he charges the public for a drug.

There may, however, be cases where the pharmacist would agree to accept the program payment plus the co-payment amount from the beneficiary as full payment, at least in instances where the covered drug is prescribed by generic name. Beneficiaries could be furnished with lists of pharmacies where such agreements were in effect.

Several other limitations on program payment appear to be feasible.

These include: a requirement, similar to that in present law with respect to Part A benefits, that in agreeing to participate in the program, the drug vendor would have to agree not to charge beneficiaries for any amounts that the Medicare program was liable for, or could be liable for; a requirement that, with respect to those prescriptions which fell at or below the co-insurance amount, the vendor would agree that the "reasonable drug charge" would be the amount at which the drug was customarily made available to the general public; and a requirement that the vendor would agree not to charge a beneficiary, with respect to any covered drug, an amount which, when added to the beneficiary co-payment and the program payment, resulted in a sum in excess of the customary charge at which the drug was available to the general public at the time the drug was furnished to the beneficiary.

CHAPTER 17
ORGANIZATION OF HEW PHARMACEUTICAL ACTIVITIES

The Department of Health, Education, and Welfare recognizes the substantial obligations it bears as a consequence of (a) the importance of prescription drugs to the health of all Americans, (b) the potential hazard to the health of individuals taking drugs, (c) the substantial cost of drugs purchased by individuals directly and through governmental programs, and (d) the economic investments that the drug firms have made to develop the capabilities they now possess. In discharging its responsibilities, the Department is mindful of its simultaneous obligations:

- To ensure that the drugs that are marketed are pure, safe, and efficacious for those who depend on them.
- To assure the continuing availability of effective drugs in adequate supply at reasonable prices and thus to promote the Nation's health.
- To encourage those firms that have invested their resources in the development, production, and distribution of drugs to persist in efforts to carry on their business, in ways that contribute increasingly to assure the quality of currently available drugs, and the continued discovery, development, testing, production, and distribution of significantly new and improved drugs.

- To carry on the research required to develop scientific knowledge essential for speeding drug development.
- To improve the quality of health care available to all Americans and, to this end, to encourage the rational prescribing of drugs.
- To stimulate the development of the needed scientific manpower (e.g., pharmacologists, toxicologists, and pharmacists).

In earlier reports of the Task Force, attention was directed to those aspects of drug research, manufacture, promotion, prescribing, and use which are largely the responsibility of the private sector, and its recommendations were directed toward increasing the mobilization of Federal resources to solve longstanding problems in these areas. While this section reaffirms the need for a community of interest, its findings and recommendations are concerned with those drug research and regulatory activities of the Federal Government which are largely intramural.

Appraisal of Organization

Recognition of both the concerns of drug users and the economic stakes of drug makers and distributors prompted the Secretary to state in his report to the President on the organization of health activities (June 1968) that he intended:

> "to examine the Department's activities in the pharmaceutical field and to determine what, if any, further reorganization is warranted."

This step was planned in order to achieve these ends:

- Determine whether like or related pharmaceutical activities could be more efficiently interrelated.
- Reassess the logic of administering food and drug regulation activities within the same agency.
- Consider how an improved scientific base could be provided for the regulation of the testing, evaluation, manufacture, distribution, and promotion of pharmaceuticals.
- Appraise the existing statutory basis for drug regulation.

As a basis for considering these issues, this chapter defines and categorizes all "pharmaceutical activities" that are carried on within the Department of Health, Education, and Welfare, indicates the magnitude of those activities and their current organizational location throughout the Department, and presents proposals to meet each of the four objectives posed above.

Definition of Pharmaceutical Activities

The Department of Health, Education, and Welfare is at one and the same time one of the Nation's largest direct and indirect purchasers of drugs, a principal stimulus for the development of new knowledge on drugs and biologicals, a principal agency for the testing of drugs, and the regulator with authority to ensure that drugs are manufactured, distributed, and promoted in compliance with the requirements of existing statutes. This substantial range of responsibilities includes the following:

Research and the Promotion of Research

- The screening of synthetic chemicals and natural products for types of pharmacological activity and the developing of those agents determined to be useful as therapeutic agents, particularly by the National Institutes of Health (NIH).
- The screening and development of psycho-pharmaceuticals within the National Institute of Mental Health (NIMH).
- The study of the interaction of environmental agents with man by the Division of Environmental Health Sciences of the NIH.
- The development of specially trained manpower and new knowledge in the fields of pharmacology-toxicology through efforts of the National Institute of General Medical Sciences and other institutes of NIH, and the support of medical, pharmacy and related institutions by the Bureau of Health Manpower.
- The review by the Food and Drug Administration (FDA) and the Division of Biologics Standards (DBS) of research conducted by drug and biological manufacturers in connection with the investigation of new drugs.
- The study of drug actions and interactions and of the biological equivalency of drugs, and the development of appropriate analytical methodology by the FDA.

Regulation

- Approval of the manufacture and distribution of new drugs, the certification of drugs containing insulin, the certification of antibiotics, the designation of official names for drugs, and the registration of producers and certain wholesalers of drugs by FDA.

- Maintenance of a drug control system by FDA that involves (a) the inspection of manufacturing facilities, (b) routine sampling of drugs on the market, (c) the control of the advertising and other promotion of drugs to prescribers, (d) the surveillance of labeling of over-the-counter drugs to ensure that it includes adequate directions for use and any necessary warnings or precautions, and (e) the continuing assembly of reports concerning adverse reactions and their analysis.
- Licensing of biological products and of manufacturers of such products by DBS.

Gathering, Processing and Dissemination of Scientific Information

- Making drug information available to consumers in the form of the package inserts and monitoring by FDA of the dissemination of this information through promotion to physicians.
- Making available current drug information through the Drug Literature Program and the Toxicology Information Program of the National Library of Medicine.
- Provision of informational support for the poison control centers throughout the nation by the Consumer Protection and Environmental Health Service.
- Development and dissemination of psycho-pharmaceutical information by the NIMH.
- Assembly of drug information and information on adverse drug reactions by the FDA as a basis for its regulatory operations.

In addition there are within the Department other activities which are closely related (by function, by techniques or facilities used, or by organizational location) to those listed above. These include the following:

- Maintenance of a network of poison control centers, the collection of data through these centers, the support of research on poisoning treatment problems and related activities by the Division of Poison Control of the Bureau of Medicine, FDA.

- Establishment of safe tolerances for pesticide residues in or on foods and the review of labeling and medical hazards to operators and eventual users of pesticides, by the Bureau of Medicine, FDA.
- Development of standards for food by the Bureau of Science, FDA.
- Establishment of standards for the quality of water by the Environmental Control Administration, CPEHS.

This report is concerned with the interrelationship of each of these several activities and assesses the effectiveness of their present organizational location within the Department. It is not concerned with the organization of those units of the Department responsible for (a) the financing of the purchase of drugs under Medicare or Medicaid, the health-related programs of the Children's Bureau, or the direct health care programs of the Health Services and Mental Health Administration; or (b) the support of research and development in pharmaceuticals through grants to nongovernmental agencies.

Magnitude and Dispersion

The foregoing categorization provides part of the factual understanding for assessment of logic with which pharmaceutical activities are distributed throughout the Department. To add perspective, and to indicate the balance or relative emphasis which may warrant attention, data are summarized here on (a) the annual expenditure in support of these activities by each organizational subdivision, and (b) the personnel utilized.

In total, the Department's annual expenditure for pharmaceutical activities will approximate $123.5 million in fiscal year 1968 and $133 million in fiscal year 1969. The makeup of this total expenditure is shown in Table 3.

Of this amount approximately:

- 64 percent, or approximately $85 million, will be devoted to the support of research and development;
- 2 percent, or approximately $3 million, will be used for the collection, organization, and dissemination of relevant information to all who use drugs, prescribe them, or market them to other manufacturers;
- 24 percent, or approximately $32.4 million, will be spent for regulatory activities; and

- 10 percent, or approximately $12.8 million, will be spent for standard-setting and control activities.

Because many health agency staff members devote their time to two or more related fields of pharmaceutical activity, it is not possible to give a precise statement of the individuals whose time and energies are now expended in each of the categories listed here. In general, however, approximately 3,740 individuals were employed in the conduct of "pharmaceutical activities" as of September 1, 1968. This total number of employees was distributed among major organizational units as follows:

NIH		560
HSMHA [b]		190
CPEHS		
FDA	2,590	
ECA	400	2,990
		3,740

[b] The pertinent number of employees in NIMH is not readily identifiable.

Influencing Factors

In appraising the organization of "pharmaceutical activities" throughout the Department, consideration must be given to a number of external factors that vitally affect the effectiveness with which departmental agencies carry on basic activities. These factors include:

The substantial and still growing dependence of the drug industry on research for the development of new drugs. This dependence creates a need for a strong research counterpart in the Federal Government that identifies areas of need and opportunity, stimulates experimentation, and collaborates with drug manufacturers in screening and appraising prospective new drugs.

The essential separateness of the Department's two basic pharmaceutical activities. The Department simultaneously (a) stimulates and promotes drug research and development as part of its total health research effort, and (b) regulates the manufacture, marketing, and promotion of drugs. These functions involve contrasting relations with private drug manufacturers which require performance by separate and independent agencies, under common and coordinating leadership.

TABLE 3. Annual Expenditures for Pharmaceutical Activities of the Department of Health, Education, and Welfare.

| | 1965 | | 1968 | | 1969[a] | |
Agency	Grants & Program Contracts	Direct Optns	Grants & Program Contracts	Direct Optns	Grants & Program Contracts	Direct Optns
National Institutes of Health: [b] [c]	(in thousands)					
NIAID	$ 2,100	$ 4,400	$ 2,500	$ 7,100	$ 2,600	$ 7,200
NCI	22,700	2,220	19,620	2,630	19,620	2,630
NINDB	10,500	----	13,490	----	14,070	----
NHI	447	129	3,820	780	3,820	780
NICH&HD	183	59	543	100	1,455	125
NIGMS	6,105	559	12,087	1,044	14,000	1,495
DRFR	----	----	993	----	1,560	----
DEHS	----	----	25	----	25	----
NLM	----	----	374	778	1,044	408
DBS	----	4,969	----	8,649	----	8,499
National Institute of Mental Health [c]	7,068	180	8,147	200	8,150	210
Food and Drug Administration [c]	----	17,141	2,817	26,188	3,175	29,493
Related Activities–						
Poison Control	50	363	269	181	279	282
Pesticides	N/A	2,291	4,369	3,376	4,714	3,223
Food	N/A	1,289	803	2,671	574	3,701
Total	$ 49,153	$ 33,600	$ 69,857	$ 53,697	$ 75,086	$ 58,046

[a] As submitted in the President's budget, January 1968.

[b] Other Institutes of the NIH expend moneys for the development and screening of drugs as an integral part of their health research efforts. It has not been possible to distinguish these expenditures from those made for the research activities to which they contribute.

[c] NIH, National Institutes of Health; NIAID, National Institute of Allergy and Infectious Diseases; NCI, National Cancer Institute; NINDB, National Institute of Neurological Diseases and Blindness; NHI, National Heart Institute; NICH&HD, National Institute of Child Health & Human Development; NIGMS, National Institute of General Medical Services; DRFR, Division of Research Facilities and Resources; DEHS, Division of Environmental Health Sciences; NLM, National Library of Medicine; DBS, Division of Biologics Standards; NIMH, National Institute of Mental Health; FDA, Food and Drug Administration.

The shortage of professionally trained scientists with the unique combinations of skills required for the Department's regulatory activity. There is no present source from which can be recruited an adequate and growing supply of physicians equipped for and interested in "regulatory medicine," i.e., dedicated to the protection of the public health through the rigorous, scientific evaluation of drugs. Simultaneously, there is not an adequate number of academic departments of clinical pharmacology to supply the skilled personnel needed for all Departmental activities, and on which the FDA can depend for a continuing supply of needed talent.

The relative external prestige of the health research and the regulatory activities of the Department. The life-saving and life-lengthening promise and results of health research endow the activities with public goodwill. That goodwill has been multiplied by imaginative and highly effective professional performance. On the other hand, the repressive, limiting character of regulatory–and, to a lesser degree, of control activities–provokes irritation, criticism, and resentment by those whose operations are affected, particularly those who violate the statutes. These underlying characteristics vitally affect the relative ability of the health research (NIH) and the regulatory (FDA) agencies of the Department to attract and hold well qualified scientific personnel for the performance of these functions.

Assessment of the Need for Change

In the light of understanding of the variety and magnitude of the pharmaceutical activities being carried on by the Department of Health, Education, and Welfare, and their functional relationship to other health care or consumer protection activities of the Department, these questions are pertinent:

- What regrouping or transfer of activities would make for their more effective administration?
- Would separation of the drug activities from other activities of the Food and Drug Administration make for their more effective administration?

As a part of the analysis underlying the reorganization of all health activities of the Department, careful consideration has already been given to the desirable organizational location of a number of activities closely related in varying degrees to activities of the Food and Drug Administration. This consideration has resulted in transfer of a number of activities previously carried on by the Bureaus of Health Services and Disease Prevention and Environmental Control of the Public Health Service to the Food and Drug Administration within the newly established Consumer Protection and Environmental Health Service. These include shellfish sanitation; pesticide label review, pesticide community studies and pesticide research; and poison control and the product-safety aspects of existing injury control programs.

Consideration is being given to the transfer of additional activities to the FDA–food protection, food sanitation research and food hazards surveillance, the regulation of food handling on interstate carriers, milk sanitation, and milk sanitation research.

These several moves would constitute a significant step toward the more efficient and economical interrelationship of activities of the Department which can use common staffs, facilities or techniques, or deal with identical or related constituencies.

The inquiry on which this report is based has focused particularly on what has been defined as "pharmaceutical activities." Analyses of these pharmaceutical activities make manifest that they are vital parts of the Department's efforts to improve the health and the environment of the American people.

> *On the basis of numerous considerations, the Task Force finds that no gain–and a substantial loss–in operating effectiveness would result from the organizational association of all pharmaceutical and related activities.*

> *More specifically, we find that:*

> *The drug development and screening programs of the National Institutes are integral parts of the biomedical research effort of the NIH and should remain the responsibility of these respective units.*

> *The manpower development activities of the NIGMS (support of the pharmacology-toxicology centers) and of the Bureau of Health Manpower of the NIH are logical parts of the total responsibilities of these two units. Transfer of these activities to related activities of the FDA would not yield adequate benefits to warrant such an organizational change. The pharmaceutical-related activities of the Bureau of Health Manpower should be administered as part of the total effort to expand needed health manpower by that bureau.*

> *The gathering, processing and dissemination of scientific information by the Consumer Protection and Environmental Health Service and its constituent, the Food and Drug Administration; by the National Library of Medicine; and by the National Institute of Mental Health are in each instance activities that flow logically out of other responsibilities of these units. These informational activities should be retained in their present organization.*

The regulatory activities of the DBS are not logically a part of the biomedical research activities of the NIH. The DBS, however, does carry on research and drug development activities related to the central functions of the NIH, and it benefits materially from association with the research staffs of several Institutes of the NIH. Some advantages would be gained by associating the regulatory activities of DBS with those of FDA. The DBS needs at times the regulatory skills of the FDA. But such transfer of the regulatory activities of DBS from NIH would result in the undesirable dissociation of these regulatory activities from the supporting research activities of NIH, and would cause a substantial loss in morale and probably a loss in key professional personnel. For these reasons, this action is not recommended.

Food and Drug Activities of FDA. History and operating practicalities have shaped the organization of the Food and Drug Administration whereby it carries on a spectrum of regulatory, control and promotional activities dealing with foods and food additives, cosmetics and therapeutic devices, and hazardous household substances as well as drugs. The original Pure Food and Drug Act established functions common to foods and to drugs that logically and economically were administered by the same agency.

Since this agency was established, and particularly during the 1960's, important changes have taken place:

- The drug activities of the FDA have been greatly expanded, particularly as a consequence of the Kefauver-Harris Amendments of 1962.
- The number and variety of drugs subject to regulation has substantially increased.
- The technology involved in the assessment of drugs has markedly advanced.

Together these factors prompt consideration of the desirability of separating drug activities from other activities of the FDA and establishing a separate agency for drug regulation and research.

In appraising this proposal, it is necessary to consider the existing internal structure of the FDA. The staffs that make up the FDA–those that handle drug activities and those that handle activities incident to the regulation of foods, food additives and cosmetics–are intermixed in each bureau in varying degrees; and often the same staff is engaged in both types of activities. The following data suggest the degree of intermixture and the nature of the dissolution required if this proposal were adopted.

		Approximate Portion of Activity[a]	
Subdivision of FDA[b]	Food	Drugs	Other
Bureau of Medicine	0.5%	94.5%	5.0%
Bureau of Veterinary Medicine	18.8	81.2	0.0
Bureau of Science	71.5	22.3	6.2
Bureau of Regulatory Compliance	46.1	46.1	7.8
Bureau of Voluntary Compliance	51.8	41.2	7.0
District Offices	56.0	[c]38.2	5.8

[a] Based on judgments of FDA administrative staff and analysis of budget.
[b] Organizational structure as of June 15, 1968.
[c] This proportion has increased markedly in recent years; estimated approximately 50 percent in 1969.

Further examination indicates that while the internal structure of each of these bureaus would permit separation of the drug activities within the Bureaus of Science, Regulatory Compliance and Voluntary Compliance, in each instance this would cause some loss in current effectiveness and some duplication of effort in the separated agencies. Within the District Offices, which represent 50 percent of the total personnel of the FDA, the staffs are substantially involved in both food and drug activities, utilize common laboratory equipment and facilities, and could not be separated without substantial duplication of staff and facilities.

In summary, the activities involved in the regulation of food, of cosmetics and of drugs–and particularly the field investigatory activities–are carried on by the same or closely related staffs. Neither the food nor the drug activities now intermixed in the FDA can, in the short run, be economically dissected out of the District Offices and administered separately.

The Task Force finds, therefore, that no clearly apparent benefits could be derived from the separation of drug regulatory activities from food regulatory activities that would offset the economy and efficiency now achieved through the maintenance of closely related investigatory, research, and regulatory staffs.

We therefore recommend that the present complex of activities now assigned to the Food and Drug Administration should continue to be administered by that agency.

Survey of Drug Prices

Increasingly, it has become apparent that the Department has an unavoidable responsibility for the continuing surveillance of drug prices because these prices are of vital concern to consumers. Included would be the accumulation of all available information on the prices of drugs, the analyses of existing indices of drug prices, the integration of drug price data–both wholesale and retail–derived by all agencies of the Department that develop or receive these data, the dissemination of information on drug prices and the results of drug price analyses, and from time to time, as circumstances make necessary, the formulation and recommendation of legislation to ensure the improved availability of drugs.

This responsibility stems from both the Department's concern that needed drugs shall be available to those consumers whose well-being depends upon them, and its responsibility for the direct or indirect expenditure (under Medicare and Medicaid) of very large sums for drugs.

At present, the responsibility for this continuing surveillance of drug prices is not fixed in any organizational unit of the Department. The Office of the Assistant Secretary for Planning and Evaluation discharged a related responsibility in 1967 in preparing its "Report on Medical Prices." The Food and Drug Administration has a clearly implied obligation under existing legislation to see to it in the interest of the consumer that "honesty and fair dealing" prevails. If authorized by the Congress, it will produce a compendium of drugs including data on the price of each drug listed. It might therefore logically assume the responsibility for the surveillance of prices as related to other responsibilities it now discharges. The National Center for Health Services Research and Development includes a small unit of economic analysts which has carried on analyses of drug prices along with other economic analyses. Both the Social and Rehabilitation Service, because of its responsibility for coordinating the administration of Medicaid by the State governments, and the Social Security Administration, because of its responsibility for the administration of Medicare, also might be charged with responsibility for the surveillance of drug prices.

Because the Social Security Administration has a clear concern with the prices of drugs, and possesses staffs most readily expandable to assume this responsibility, we recommend that the Social Security Administration should undertake continuing responsibility for the surveillance of drug costs, average prescription prices, and drug use.

If the SSA is assigned such responsibility, those individuals on the staff of the National Center for Health Services Research and Development now engaged in the accumulation of data on the cost of drugs should be transferred to the Social Security Administration. The Social and Rehabilitation Service must continue to maintain a small staff responsible for assisting the State governments in the purchase of drugs by the accumulation of data and analyses of the States' experience in the purchase, use, and cost of drugs.

Improvement of Scientific Capability

If, as is proposed, no substantial organizational change is made, there will remain the urgent need to improve the scientific capability of the staff responsible for drug regulation. This important need grows out of the substantial expansion of FDA's responsibilities for drug regulation within recent years and the difficulties encountered in recruiting qualified professional personnel. To meet this need, the FDA has taken significant steps to:

- Attract more and better qualified professional personnel, particularly physicians, by making employment arrangements more attractive, by developing orientation programs to acquaint those who are recruited with the full panoply of the Department's pharmaceutical activities, by (a) offering individuals opportunities for simultaneous clinical and/or research experience, while serving the FDA, and (b) providing leaves of absence for educational and research assignments.
- Supplement the capabilities of the FDA's in-house staff by contracting with medical schools throughout the country (as has been done with the Georgetown Medical School) and by seeking ways of making fuller use of the Public Health Service hospitals for supportive clinical research.

Immediate Opportunities. These steps alone are not enough. The critical nature of the problem of enhancing the scientific capabilities of

FDA's staff is made more pressing by the necessity of (a) acting upon the recommendations of the NAS-NRC drug study, and (b) finding replacements for those physicians who were assigned by the PHS to assist the FDA and whose assignments are now being completed.

We therefore recommend that efforts should be strengthened to assure that the skills of experts both within and outside of the Department of Health, Education, and Welfare are used to augment the scientific capabilities of the Food and Drug Administration.

This might be accomplished, in part, by enlisting the assistance of individual scientists from health agencies within the Federal Government to serve for limited periods on tasks which they deemed relevant to their research interests, or by their acceptance of *ad hoc* assignments for the evaluation of specific drugs or other priority work.

In addition, the Commissioner of Food and Drugs should strengthen the efforts to establish a full and continuing association of the Food and Drug Administration with the Nation's medical schools, pharmacy schools, and the biomedical scientific community. This might include contracting with relevant specialists on the staffs of the five medical school faculties in the Washington area to assist with the review of Investigational New Drug exemptions (IND's) and New Drug Applications (NDA's).

These efforts should also include the substantial expansion of the current use of advisory committees. It is particularly proposed that the FDA be directed to explore the feasibility of establishing a series of *ad hoc* panels made up of the best relevant medical and scientific talent throughout the country to assist with the review of IND's and NDA's for all new chemical entities or other drugs submitted for approval.

Review of IND data and NDA's by personnel outside FDA would pose problems concerning the maintenance of the confidentiality of material submitted for review by drug manufacturers. We believe, however, that adequate safeguards can be established to ensure the protection of the interests of the manufacturers. The value to be derived from the association of the FDA staff with outstanding talent throughout the country, i.e., the enrichment of the experience of staff personnel and the authoritativeness added to FDA decisions made after consultation with such panels, would be so great as to warrant an early and substantial effort to bring these panels into being.

Long-Range Opportunities. In addition, three alternative proposals for enhancing the scientific capability of the FDA's drug evaluation staff have been considered. These proposals are as follows:

1. A "Therapeutic Appeals Board" should be established within (or without) NIH to provide both scientific and clinical capabilities, supplementing those possessed by the FDA. It would be provided with staff and facilities to carry on basic research and clinical studies through association with both Federal and non-Federal health facilities. These facilities would be utilized to study and evaluate selected drugs submitted by manufacturers or by the FDA, when an NDA has been refused approval by the FDA.
2. An Institute of Pharmacology should be established within the NIH to carry on research in the field underlying the regulatory function of the FDA and to administer the program of support for the pharmacology-toxicology centers.
3. A clinical and laboratory facility should be established within the FDA to concentrate on research concerned with the use, efficacy, and toxicity of drugs, and the development of new methods and approaches to their evaluation. It would provide opportunities within FDA for a continuum of research and application extending from molecular pharmacology through animal testing to clinical experience.

Such a center could pursue a multi-disciplinary approach combining the efforts of pharmacologists, toxicologists, clinical investigators, biochemists, experimental pathologists, medicinal chemists, geneticists and perhaps others. It would require laboratory and clinical facilities. And it would need to have an effective system of communication with several institutes of the NIH, and particularly with the National Institute of General Medical Sciences and the pharmacology-toxicology centers which that institute supports.

A Choice Among Alternatives. Each of these alternative proposals would provide supplementary laboratory and clinical research facilities and thus enhance the existing capabilities of the Bureau of Medicine of the FDA by:

- Strengthening the scientific aspects of drug evaluation, and probably modernizing methods; and
- Attracting (in various degrees) a greater number of men and women possessing medical and scientific competence to these activities.

The alternatives differ in that (a) the "Therapeutic Board" would combine research and appeal responsibilities, (b) the Institute of Pharmacology within NIH would have both a research and a manpower function, and (c) the FDA drug research facility would provide a broadly based research effort.

But each of the first two proposals would separate drug research activities from drug regulation activities. Such organizational separation would establish an artificial and unnatural divergence between the agency responsible for fact finding and the agency responsible for acting on those facts.

The proposal for a "Therapeutic Appeals Board" poses an added organizational handicap. Acceptance of this proposal would establish a supplementary capability, of necessarily limited competence, and, by providing an added appeals opportunity for drug manufacturers, would undermine the regulatory strength of the FDA.

Establishment of a research capability within NIH, i.e., the establishment of an Institute of Pharmacology, would "borrow" from the competence, reputation, and prestige of that agency to increase the capability of FDA. It would, however, be an illogical organizational arrangement within the NIH; pharmacology is, among other things, a tool discipline used by many or all existing institutes, and all research in or use of this discipline cannot properly be concentrated in a new and separate institute. Moreover, establishment of such an institute would give no assurance of better relating the NIH capabilities with the needs of FDA–a notable lack to date. The use of relevant experts on the NIH staffs to assist FDA on specific problems in which they have a special interest and competence offers a greater likelihood of making NIH's substantial capabilities available to the FDA, and accordingly "separate" capability will be less needed.

In the long run, it is essential that the capability of the Bureau of Medicine itself be increased both by (a) the upgrading of the existing medical staff and (b) the inclusion in this Bureau of supplementary scientific personnel equipped with the facilities needed for carrying on relevant research.

Because it constitutes the preferable means for creating the additional scientific capability that is required, the Task Force recommends that legislation should be enacted to authorize establishment within the Food and Drug Administration of a clinical and laboratory facility to provide the necessary

opportunities for research by highly qualified basic scientists and clinicians.

In recognition of the substantial contributions of the late Senator Royal S. Copeland toward enactment of the present Food, Drug and Cosmetic Act, we propose that this facility be known as the Royal S. Copeland Research Center.

Reappraisal of Drug Evaluation Methods

In addition to increasing the scientific capability of the regulatory staffs, there is need for reappraising the relevance and efficiency of methods now used by DBS and FDA to evaluate the safety and effectiveness of pharmaceuticals.

Three methods are now used:

1. The approval of new drug applications by FDA is substantially an assessment of the research evidence presented in support of the safety and effectiveness of pharmaceuticals. It also includes a critical evaluation of manufacturing facilities and verification of the strength, quality and purity of drugs and of the proposed manufacturing and control procedures. The approval granted for the distribution of a new drug may be withdrawn for cause.
2. The certification of antibiotics and insulin by FDA involves initial approval by the methods described in the preceding paragraph, and in addition, the analysis of every production batch before distribution. Batches which do not comply with applicable regulations are denied certification, and cannot be distributed legally. Certification may be discontinued at any time if conditions of certification are violated.
3. The approval of biologicals by DBS involves the licensing of both the establishment and the product, and the subsequent review of control protocols and/or continuing study of samples.

These methods are now founded in legislation as well as in historical practice. Yet the logic or necessity of these methods is subject to substantial and widespread questioning, and their suitability deserves careful examination.

To help assure the uniform high quality of drugs marketed in interstate commerce, the Task Force earlier recommended consideration of a licensing and registration system for drugs and drug producers. The favorable experience of DBS and of pharmaceutical control authorities in other countries suggests that such a system can also be used for the evaluation and premarketing clearance of new drugs.

The Task Force therefore recommends that the Secretary of Health, Education, and Welfare should, after consultation with representatives of the drug industry, pharmacy, clinical medicine, and consumer groups, should appoint a study group to reappraise the efficiency of methods now used by the Division of Biologics Standards and the Food and Drug Administration to evaluate the safety and effectiveness of pharmaceuticals. The participants should direct attention to the appropriateness of the three existing classifications of pharmaceuticals–new drugs and "not new" drugs, certifiable products, and biologics. The study group should also consider the feasibility of developing a registration and licensing system which would assure that all drugs marketed in interstate commerce are produced under adequate quality control standards.

Consideration of such a system will inevitably involve a simultaneous assessment of the combined industry-government effort to discover new drugs and to bring them promptly from the research laboratory to the patient. The effectiveness of this combined effort requires, on the one hand, that the research conducted by industry and the reports of this research submitted as a basis for the approval of the FDA and DBS be thorough, competent and persistently reliable; and, on the other hand, that the review of these research reports by the scientists of FDA and DBS be equally thorough, competent and reliable.

CONSULTANTS AND WORKSHOP PARTICIPANTS

During the 20 months of its operations, the Task Force and the Task Force Staff were particularly fortunate in having the advice, guidance, support and criticism of more than 160 nongovernmental experts representing clinical medicine, pharmacology, pharmacy, medical and pharmacy schools, professional health organizations, drug manufacturing, drug distribution, health insurance, data processing, economics, law, and a variety of consumer groups.

Some of these individuals served as formal consultants to the Task Force, others served informally, and still others participated in workshops and other Task Force conferences. Many of them gave generously of weeks or months of their time, providing assistance which was invaluable to the Task Force in its work.

Similar and equally valuable assistance was provided by many members of State and Federal agencies who worked closely with the Task Force. Among them were representatives of the Departments of Commerce, Defense, Labor, Justice and Treasury, the Office of Economic Opportunity, and the Veterans Administration, and especially members of American Embassy staffs in foreign countries who aided in the collection of much previously unavailable data on foreign drug programs.

The contributions of all of these are gratefully acknowledged. They have no responsibility, however, for any technical errors in any of the Task Force publications, nor for any conclusions reached by the Task Force.

Their listing here in no way suggests that any of them have approved or disapproved the Task Force findings and recommendations.

Although it is impossible to list all those who participated, and apologies are proffered to those whose names may have been inadvertently omitted, particular thanks are extended to the following:

Morris Aarons
General Counsel and Executive Secretary
National Association of Pharmaceutical
Manufacturers

Brian Abel-Smith
Professor of Social Administration
London (England) School of Economics

Edward S. Albers, Jr.
President
Albers Drug Company

M. G. Allmark
Assistant Director General
Food and Drug Directorate, Canada

Betty Jane Anderson
American Medical Association

Mary Louise Anderson
Chairman, House of Delegates
American Pharmaceutical Association

William S. Apple, Ph.D.
Executive Director
American Pharmaceutical Association

Sydney Aronson, President
Paid Prescriptions, Inc.

Karl Bambach, Ph.D., Consultant
Pharmaceutical Manufacturers Association

Joseph Barrows, Past President
National Association of Pharmaceutical
Manufacturers

Patrick Benner
Assistant Secretary Supply Division
Ministry of Health, Great Britain

Robert Berson, M.D.
Executive Director
Association of American Medical Colleges

Karl H. Beyer, Jr., M.D., Ph.D.
Senior Vice President
Merck, Sharp & Dohme Research Laboratories

Howard Binkley, Vice President,
Administration and Planning
Pharmaceutical Manufacturers Association

William E. Bittle
Statistician
Communications Workers of America

Charles W. Bliven, Ph.D.
Executive Secretary
American Association of Colleges of Pharmacy

Robert J. Bolger
Executive Vice President
National Association of Chain Drug Stores

Clarence Borgelt
Toledo Health and Retirees Center
American Federation of Labor–Council of
Industrial Organization

Irwin Breslow, M.D.
Director of Clinical Pharmacology
Graduate Hospital
University of Pennsylvania

J. L. Broadbent, M.D.
Senior Medical Officer
Committee on the Safety of Drugs
Ministry of Health, Great Britain

Donald C. Brodie, Ph.D.
Associate Dean
School of Pharmacy
University of California

B. H. Brooks
Department of External Affairs
New Zealand

Stanley F. Buch
Buch's Pharmacy
Lancaster, Pa.

Oliver H. Buchanan, Ph.D.
Professor of Information Science
Pratt Institute, NYC

John Burns, M.D.
Director of Medical Research
Hoffman-LaRoche Company

Richard Burr
R. A. Gosselin and Co., Inc.
Dedham, Mass.

Roger Cain
Executive Secretary
American College of Apothecaries

Herbert S. Carlin
Associate Professor and Director
Hospital Pharmacy Service
Medical Center
University of Illinois

Blue A. Carstenson
Assistant Director of Legislative Services
National Farmers Union

R. A. Chapman, Ph.D.
Director General
Food and Drug Directorate, Canada

Ronald Clark
Head, Industry Affairs
Smith Kline & French Laboratories, Ltd.,
England

Charles B. Cleveland
Manager of Science Information
Pharmaceutical Manufacturers Association

Leighton Cluff, M.D.
Chairman, Department of Medicine
College of Medicine
University of Florida

Theodore Colton, Sc.D.
Associate Professor of Biostatistics
Harvard Medical School

E. T. Conybeare, M.D.
Head, Special Medical Services "A"
Ministry of Health, Great Britain

Chauncey I. Cooper
Dean, College of Pharmacy
Howard University

John J. Corson
Consultant to the Secretary
U.S. Department of Health, Education,
and Welfare

Melvin Crotty
Central Pharmaceutical Service
Washington, D.C.

John J. Curry, M.D.
Council on Drugs
American Medical Association

Roy C. Darlington, Ph.D.
Professor, College of Pharmacy
Howard University

W. Palmer Dearing, President
Group Health Association of America

Paul de Haen
Paul de Haen, Inc.

Nils Äke Diding, M.D.
Director, Apotekens Central Laboratorium
Solna, Sweden

Durwood F. Dodgen
Assistant Director of the Scientific Division
American Pharmaceutical Association

Harry F. Dowling, M.D.
Head of the Department of Medicine
University of Illinois College of Medicine

Frederick Elliott, M.D.
American Hospital Association

Dorothy Ellsworth
Special Representative
Brotherhood of Railway Clerks

Medicinalradet Folke Ernerfeldt
National Board of Health
Sweden

Karl Evang, M.D.
Director General of Health
Norway

E. Fawcitt
Deputy Chief Pharmacist
Ministry of Health, Great Britain

Edward Feldman, Ph.D.
Director, National Formulary
American Pharmaceutical Association

William C. Fitch
Executive Director
American Association of Retired Persons

John Fleming
Pension Welfare Department
American Bakery and Confectionery
Workers Union

Joseph F. Follman, Jr.
Director of Information and Research
Health Insurance Association of America

William L. Ford
Executive Vice President
National Wholesale Druggists' Association

Marlane C. Gainor
School of Pharmacy
University of Pittsburgh

Melvin A. Glasser
Director, Social Security Department
United Auto Workers of America

Sir George Godber
Chief Medical Officer
Ministry of Health, Great Britain

Stuart Gold, Project Director,
National Disease and Therapeutic Index
Lea Associates

Avram Goldstein, M.D.
Professor of Pharmacology
School of Medicine
Stanford University

Jere E. Goyan, Ph.D.
Dean, School of Pharmacy
University of California

George B. Griffenhagen
Director of Communications
American Pharmaceutical Association

Harry Harley, M.D., Chairman,
Committee on Drug Costs and Prices
House of Commons, Canada, 1967

Stephen Harris
Industrial Union Department
American Federation of Labor–Council of
Industrial Organization

Henry H. Harvey
Assistant Director of Professional Relations
Blue Cross Association

James G. Haughton, M.D.
First Deputy Administrator
Health Services Administration
New York City

Thomas Hayes, M.D.
Director, Department of Drugs
American Medical Association

Hans Hellberg, Director
State Pharmaceutical Laboratory of Sweden

William Heller, Ph.D.
United States Pharmacopeia

Elmer C. Hillman, Jr., Member
Professional Relations Committee
National Association of Chain Drug Stores

John L. S. Holloman, Jr., M.D.
Past President
National Medical Association

Alfred W. Hubbard, Editor
Modern Medicine Publications, Inc.

William Hutton, Executive Director
National Council of Senior Citizens

Raymond Jang, Consultant
American Society of Hospital Pharmacists

Hershel Jick, M.D., Director
Clinical Pharmacology Laboratory
Lemuel Shattuck Hospital
Jamaica Plain, Mass.

Edwin Jordan, M.D.
Executive Director
American Association of Medical Clinics

Guy R. Justus, Director
American Public Welfare Association

Louis E. Kazin, Editor
National Association of Retail Druggists
Journal

Lorin E. Kerr, M.D.
Assistant to the Executive Medical Officer
United Mine Workers Welfare
and Retirement Fund

Harry A. Kimbriel
Executive Vice President
National Wholesale Druggist Association

Jan Koch-Weser, M.D.
Director, Clinical Pharmacology Unit
Massachusetts General Hospital

Louis Lasagna, M.D.
Professor of Medicine and Pharmacology
School of Medicine
Johns Hopkins University

Armistead Lee
Director of Economic Research
Pharmaceutical Manufacturers Association

Leonard Lesser
Assistant to the President
Industrial Union Department
American Federation of Labor–Council
of Industrial Organization

Gerhard Levy, Ph.D.
Professor of Pharmacy
University of Buffalo

John R. Lewis, Ph.D.
Department of Drugs
American Medical Association

A. F. Liebnau
Toledo Health and Retirees Center
American Federation of Labor–Council
of Industrial Organization

Paul Lofholm
Assistant Clinical Professor
School of Pharmacy
University of California

Rune Lönngren, M.D., Chairman
Government Expert Committee on Drug
Supply and Distribution, Sweden

Fred T. Mahaffey
Executive Director and Secretary
National Association of Boards of Pharmacy

Sir Leonard Mallen, Chairman
Pharmaceutical Benefits Committee
Commonwealth of Australia

Abraham Marcus
Editor-in-Chief
International Tribune of Great Britain

Robert Maronde, M.D.
Professor of Medicine and Pharmacology
School of Medicine
University of Southern California

Arthur I. Martin
Director of Systems and Data Processing
E. R. Squibb & Sons

Christopher Martin, M.D.
Director of Georgetown Medical Program
Georgetown University

Eric W. Martin, Ph.D.
Director of Medical Communication
Lederle Laboratories

Geneva Mathiasen
Executive Director
National Council on the Aging

Margaret McCarron, M.D.
Associate Clinical Professor of Medicine
University of Southern California
School of Medicine

Joseph D. McEvilla, Ph.D.
Professor of Pharmaceutical Economics
School of Pharmacy
University of Pittsburgh

John McHugh
Director of Professional Relations
National Association of Chain Drug Stores

Walter McLean, R.Ph.
Louisiana State Department of Welfare

Robert E. McMillen, Research Director
United Association of Plumbing
and Pipe Fitting Industry

George Melcher, Jr., M.D.
President
Group Health Insurance, Inc.

Harold Meyers
Hospital Consultant
Welfare and Retirement Fund
United Mine Workers of America

Lloyd C. Miller, Ph.D.
Director of Revision
U.S. Pharmacopeia

Walter Modell, M.D.
Professor of Pharmacology
School of Medicine
Cornell University

A. B. Morrison, Ph.D.
Director, Research Laboratories
Food and Drug Directorate
Ottawa, Canada

Charlotte Muller, Ph.D.
Professor of Urban Studies
Graduate Center
The City University of New York

Harold S. Newman, M.D., Director
Group Health Cooperative of Puget Sound

Sarah Newman, General Secretary
National Consumers League

Edwin W. Nicklas, M.D.
Washington, D.C.

Joseph A. Oddis, Executive Secretary
American Society of Hospital Pharmacists

Grant Osborn, Ph.D.
Professor Insurance
University of Massachusetts

Mrs. Cynthia Palmer
Statistics Section
Ministry of Health, Great Britain

Michael L. Parker, Attorney
Landels, Ripley, Gregory & Diamond

Harold G. Pearce, Vice President
Blue Cross Association

Edmund Pellegrino, M.D.
Director, Medical Center
State University of New York
at Stoneybrook

John Preston, Ph.D., Vice President
National Pharmaceutical Council, Inc.

John H. Pruitt, Director,
Medical Services
Endicott Johnson Corporation

Robert Quinnell, M.D., Director
Office of Medical Relations
Pharmaceutical Manufacturers Association

Kenneth Reese
Contributing Editor
Chemical & Engineering News

Dan Rennick
Editor, *American Druggist*

G. Frederick Roll
Assistant to the President
Smith Kline & French Laboratories

Edward Rosenow, M.D.
Executive Director
American College of Physicians

James Russo, Director
Special Studies
Pharmaceutical Manufacturers Association

Joseph F. Sadusk, Jr., M.D.
Vice President
Parke, Davis & Company

Stanley Schor, Ph.D.
Chairman, Department of Biometrics
School of Medicine
Temple University

Leonard Schifrin, Ph.D.
Chairman, Department of Economics
College of William and Mary

George Schwartz
Sales Manager
American Pharmaceutical Company

Bert Seidman, Director
Department of Social Security
American Federation of Labor–Council
of Industrial Organization

Joseph Senturia
Industrial Relations Consultant
United Steelworkers of America

Jay R. Shapiro, M.D.
Washington, D.C.

Kenneth Shaw
International Vice President
Brotherhood of Railway Clerks

Irving Shaw, President
Vitarine Company

Harry C. Shirkey, M.D.
Medical Director
Children's Hospital
Birmingham, Ala.

Richard E. Shoemaker
Social Security Department
American Federation of Labor–
Council of Industrial Organization

William G. Shoemaker
Pharmaceutical Services Specialist
Bureau of Medical Services
Office of Public Assistance
Harrisburg, Pa.

P. Siderius, M.D.
Director-General of Health Care
The Netherlands

Abraham E. Slesser, Ph.D.
Assistant Technical Director
Smith Kline & French Laboratories

Björn Smedby, M.D., Research Associate
Department of Social Medicine
University of Uppsala, Sweden

Lawrence Smedley
Department of Social Security
American Federation of Labor–
Council of Industrial Organization

Joseph E. Snyder, M.D.
Presbyterian Hospital
Columbia Medical Center, New York

Saul Solomon, M.D.
New York Hotel Trades Council

Henry B. Steele, Ph.D.
Professor of Economics
University of Houston

C. Joseph Stetler, President
Pharmaceutical Manufacturers Association

Waldo A. Stevens
Senior Vice President, Operations
National Association of Blue Shield Plans

James Struthers, M.D.
Principal Medical Officer
Ministry of Health, Great Britain

Lars Sundin
Lakemedelsstatistik, AB, Sweden

Fred A. Tate, Ph.D., Assistant Director
Chemical Abstract Service
Chemical Abstracts Society

Norval Taylor, Medical Assessor
Committee on the Classification of
    Proprietary Preparations
Ministry of Health, Great Britain

George Teeling-Smith, Director
Office of Health Economics
Association of the British
Pharmaceutical Industry

E. B. Teesdale, Director
Association of the British
Pharmaceutical Industry

Julia Thompson
Director of the Washington Office
American Nurses' Association

Linwood F. Tice, Ph.D., Dean
Philadelphia College of Pharmacy and Science

Malcolm Tottie, M.D., Chairman
Committee on International Health Relations
National Board of Health, Sweden

Duke Trexler
Executive Secretary
National Academy of Sciences/National
Research Council

Vernon O. Trygstad, President
National Pharmaceutical Council

Harold Upjohn, M.D.
Director of Medical Research
Upjohn Company

Lawrence C. Weaver, Ph.D.
Dean, College of Pharmacy
University of Minnesota

Clayton G. Weigand, M.D.
Director of Medical Administration
Eli Lilly and Company

Julian A. Weiss
Director of Pharmaceutical Operations
Kaiser Foundation Hospitals

Isaac Welt, Ph.D., Deputy Director
Scientific & Technical Information Systems
Center for Technology and Administration
American University

Rune Westerling
Apotekarsocieteten
Stockholm, Sweden

Jean K. Weston, M.D.
Vice President
National Pharmaceutical Council

T. D. Whittet
Chief Pharmacist
Ministry of Health, Great Britain

William Wigle, M.D., President
Pharmaceutical Manufacturers of Canada

Kenneth W. Wisowaty, Director
Environmental Research and Planning
National Association of Blue Shield Plans

A. R. Wood
Second Secretary, Administration
New Zealand Embassy (Washington, D.C.)

William E. Woods
Washington Office Representative
National Association of Retail Druggists

Editor's Note

Dr. Philip Lee is Professor Emeritus of Social Medicine at the University of California-San Francisco. Along with Milton Silverman and Mia Lydecker, he is the author of a number of policy-related books, including *The Drugging of the Americas, Pills, Profits and Politics,* and *Pills & The Public Purse.*

In the following article, reprinted from the *Drug Information Journal,* Dr. Lee shares his thoughts on the work and results of the Task Force on Prescription Drugs.

[Haworth co-indexing entry note]: "Editor's Note." Smith, Mickey C. Co-published simultaneously in *Journal of Research in Pharmaceutical Economics* (Pharmaceutical Products Press, an imprint of The Haworth Press, Inc.) Vol. 10, No. 4, 2001, p. 181; and: *Prescription Drugs Under Medicare: The Legacy of the Task Force on Prescription Drugs* (ed: Mickey C. Smith) Pharmaceutical Products Press, an imprint of The Haworth Press, Inc., 2001, p. 181. Single or multiple copies of this article are available for a fee from The Haworth Document Delivery Service [1-800-342-9678, 9:00 a.m. - 5:00 p.m. (EST). E-mail address: getinfo@haworthpressinc.com].

The Task Force on Prescription Drugs:
A Review of Problems, Progress and Possibilities

Philip R. Lee

The Task Force on Prescription Drugs was established by Health, Education and Welfare (HEW) Secretary John Gardner in 1967 to undertake a comprehensive study of the problems of including the cost of prescription drugs under Medicare. The job proved far more complex and difficult than it appeared at the outset. What seemed to be an economic and political problem proved to be much more of a scientific and management problem, with implications not only for the elderly but for all taxpayers, the drug industry, insurance companies, health professionals and health care institutions, and federal and state governments.

The Task Force worked for 20 months, submitting an initial report in March 1968 and a final report in February 1969. The latter included 48 major findings, 25 recommendations, and 5 background papers on the Drug Users, Drug Prescribers, Drug Makers and Drug Distributors, Foreign Drug Programs, and Approaches to Drug Insurance Design.[1]

Philip R. Lee, M.D., is Professor of Social Medicine, University of California-San Francisco, Box 0936, 3333 California 265, San Francisco, CA 94143.

Presented at the Twelfth Annual Meeting, Drug Information Association, San Francisco, June 23-26, 1976.

Reprinted with permission from *Drug Information Journal* 1977;11(Mar):7-10.

[Haworth co-indexing entry note]: "The Task Force on Prescription Drugs: A Review of Problems, Progress and Possibilities." Lee, Philip R. Co-published simultaneously in *Journal of Research in Pharmaceutical Economics* (Pharmaceutical Products Press, an imprint of The Haworth Press, Inc.) Vol. 10, No. 4, 2001, pp. 183-191; and: *Prescription Drugs Under Medicare: The Legacy of the Task Force on Prescription Drugs* (ed: Mickey C. Smith) Pharmaceutical Products Press, an imprint of The Haworth Press, Inc., 2001, pp. 183-191.

To summarize these reports and background papers would be a formidable job. It would be even more difficult to assess their impact on the drug industry, health professions, insurance industry, federal and state governments, and consumers. Rather than attempt such a comprehensive analysis, I will focus on several of the major findings and recommendations and assess their impact.

After thorough review of the available information and the issues, the Task Force concluded that a drug insurance program under Medicare was needed by the elderly and that it would be both economically and medically feasible. Recommendation was made that such a program be instituted. In the eight years since that recommendation, repeated efforts have been made to add an outpatient drug benefit to the Medicare program, with little success. The proposals that have received the most serious consideration were designed along the lines recommended by the Task Force. Most recently, serious interest has been expressed in substantial drug coverage under a national health insurance program. In considering the design of a drug insurance system–either as an expanded Medicare benefit or as part of a national health insurance program–a number of policy decisions must be made. Before examining these policy issues, however, the potential size of the operation must be considered.

Drug therapy is by far the most widely practiced form of therapy. On the average, 1.1 prescriptions are written for every patient visit to a physician. It is estimated, for example, that some 2.8 billion prescriptions were dispensed in the United States last year at a total cost of about $14 billion. Of these, about two-thirds were dispensed by community pharmacies (independents and chains), discount stores, and dispensing physicians, and one-third by hospital pharmacies. In addition, an estimated one-half billion was spent for prescription drugs by military hospitals, VA hospitals and the Public Health Service, and roughly $4.5 billion was spent for nonprescription or over-the-counter medications.

The cost and number of prescriptions dispensed will continue to increase in the future, because of the steady rise of average prescription prices, the growing number of prescriptions per patient per year, the increase of the total population, the increased number of the elderly, and the increased incidence of chronic disease. Furthermore, judging from the experience of other programs and other countries, it is likely that drug utilization will increase by about 15 percent in the first year after a national drug insurance program goes into effect, and by smaller increments thereafter.

Designing an effective drug insurance program is not a simple business. In its final report the Task Force on Prescription Drugs considered the questions of who should be covered, what the scope of benefits should be, how the program could be financed, whether co-payments or deductibles should be used, how pharmacists should be paid, and what means of utilization review might be used. Although it looked at Medicare population only, the Task Force observed:

> Reasonable program costs appear to be associated with (a) the use of a formulary developed by or in cooperation with the medical community, (b) the use of copayment or coinsurance, (c) the use of utilization review procedures to prevent or minimize irrational prescribing, (d) the use of appropriate electronic or other data processing methods, with appropriate drug coding techniques, (e) simplified determination of beneficiary eligibility, (f) population coverage which obviates adverse selection of high risk beneficiaries, (g) the use of a vender payment formula based on actual acquisition cost verified by field audits rather than any catalogue or wholesale price list, and (h) operation with the program serving as the legal purchasing agent, with utilization of competitive and negotiated bids, rather than merely as the reimbursing group.[2]

These observations are even more important today, as we look at the problems of covering prescription drugs under national health insurance. The issue of efficient administration and how this can be achieved remains perhaps the most serious problem that must be resolved if a cost effective program is to be carried out. Time has not diminished the need of some elderly for financial aid to meet the cost of prescription drugs. It has, however, increased awareness of the complexities of designing and implementing a drug insurance program with its many administrative, economic and professional ramifications.

During the considerations of the Task Force, and increasingly since then, the following essential points have emerged:

-The major objective must be not the lowest possible cost of the drugs, but the best possible health of the patients.
-Drug prices should be kept low but they must not be reduced

to the point at which they represent a real (not a hypothetical) threat to the industry's research.

 – Reimbursement to the pharmacist must cover not only the drugs dispensed, but reasonable compensation for professional services.
 – The use of generic drug products will offer some savings, but it would be unwise to expect that these savings will be exceptionally large.
 – In any drug utilization review, major emphasis must be placed on patient benefit rather than exclusively on cost savings. Here the goal is not cheap prescribing but rational prescribing.

In the Task Force initial report, issued on March 7, 1968, the following two recommendations were included:

 – Legislation to permit the establishment of reasonable cost and charge ranges, and limits of Federal participation in reimbursement, for drugs supplied under the Medicare, Medicaid and Maternal and Child Health programs. Such ranges would not be used where hospitals and other health care institutions have already established effective and reliable systems of cost and quality control.
 – Legislation to permit the establishment of a Federal Drug Compendium, to be published and distributed to all physicians, pharmacies, hospitals and other appropriate individuals and institutions, to provide all of the necessary information in readily accessible and comprehensive form.[3]

These two recommendations received mixed reviews, and the first led to a program that has been enmeshed in controversy. In 1972, the Social Security Act Amendments included provisions for measures that would achieve economies in the Medicare and Medicaid programs. Although the focus of congressional concern was on soaring hospital costs and the rapid increase in the cost of physicians' services, one of the federal government's major moves was in the field of prescription drug costs.

Under a plan proposed by HEW, called the Maximum Allowable Cost (MAC) plan, HEW would strive to control Medicare and Medicaid drug costs by the following means:

1. Limit pharmacists' reimbursement for prescriptions to their actual acquisition cost plus a dispensing fee. Pharmacists in many state programs were found to be reimbursed on the basis of a published wholesale price which was often more than 15 percent higher than the actual acquisition cost of the drug.
2. Limit reimbursement for chemically identical drugs which are formulated by two or more manufacturers to the price of the lowest priced of those drugs generally available to pharmacists. This MAC plan would be established by a Pharmaceutical Reimbursement Board composed of government drug experts, and assisted by a nongovernment advisory panel. The Food and Drug Administration (FDA) would first review the drugs for pending regulatory problems and problems of biological equivalence.
3. Make comprehensive price information on drugs available to practicing physicians and pharmacists to enable them to consider the cost to patients. The greatest impact of this price information would probably be on privately financed prescription drug purchases rather than on government-financed programs.

The MAC program has yet [as of June 1976] to be implemented. The regulations were published in final form in July 1975 and were originally scheduled to take effect on April 26, 1976. The date was extended to August 26, 1976 in order to accommodate state Medicaid programs that were not yet ready to make the necessary changes and to give HEW more time to develop current and accurate price information.

These regulations are not a perfect instrument of public policy, but they are a measured and re[a]sonable attempt at cost constraint in a market which itself is far from perfect. It can achieve modest but significant savings without disrupting the market and without interfering in medical practice.

Not everyone agrees with HEW on the MAC program. The American Medical Association (AMA) and other medical groups have taken HEW to court on the grounds that the regulations interfere with the practice of medicine and are not authorized under the Social Security Act. The AMA has been joined by the Pharmaceutical Manufacturers Association (PMA), which argues strongly against the validity of HEW's procedures for quality and equivalence review. Most recently, the regulations have been challenged by the National Association of Retail Druggists, which questions the validity of estimated acquisition costs and the lack of national standards concerning dispensing fees. All these suits are working their way through the courts. The AMA and PMA suits are fairly well advanced and there could be some action by the court in the near future.

What happened to the idea of a Federal Drug Compendium? For the last decade, Senator Gaylord Nelson and others have introduced legislation in each Congress that would authorize publication and distribution of a compendium of prescription drugs to replace the present package inserts and, hopefully, to replace the Physicians' Desk Reference. Although the legislation has never been enacted, two years ago the FDA established a task force within the Bureau of Drugs to explore this area in depth. Perhaps this effort will provide a new approach to resolve this issue after more than ten years of discussion and debate.

Many of the recommendations of the Task Force have been implemented with far less controversy than those related to an outpatient prescription drug benefit for the elderly under Medicare, controlling the costs of drugs in federally subsidized medical care programs, and the publication of a Federal Drug Compendium. In July 1967, the Task Force initiated a series of meetings on drug classification and coding that proved highly successful. Before the Task Force finished its work a proposed classification had been developed in cooperation with representatives of the AMA, the U.S. Pharmacopeia, the National Formulary, the American Society of Hospital Pharmacists, the Drug Information Association, the National Pharmaceutical Council, the PMA, the FDA, the National Library of Medicine and various universities and state agencies. A universal coding, classification and identification system was developed as a result of these efforts. That coding system has been adopted by government and industry and it is used in the National Drug Code Directory. Since its initial adoption, it has undergone several revisions.

Drug utilization review was not a widely accepted practice in 1969 when the Task Force recommended support for "pilot research projects on prescription drug utilization review methods."[4] In 1972, without particular reference to the problems of drug utilization review, Congress amended the Social Security Act and mandated creation of Professional Standards Review Organizations (PSROs) to review the quality and necessity of medical care provided to federal beneficiaries in the Medicare, Medicaid, Crippled Childrens' and other Maternal

and Child Health programs. The PSRO system was created in light of
the past experience of county medical society-sponsored foundations
for medical care, hospital utilization review and medical audit committees, and hospital discharge data systems. The PSROs will seek to
assure the medical necessity of care primarily through a detailed process of concurrent review of inpatient hospital care. In addition to the
PSRO reviews of inpatient care, efforts have been made to carry out
drug utilization review in a variety of ambulatory care settings.

Progress has also been made in the organization of HEW pharmaceutical activities and the expansion of support for research in drug
utilization review and for training in clinical pharmacy and clinical
pharmacology. The most important organizational changes were the
transfer of the Division of Biologics Standards from the National
Institutes of Health to the FDA, and the development of the Drug
Studies Branch in the Office of Research and Statistics, Social Security Administration. Expanded support for drug utilization and related
studies have been provided by the Center for Health Services Research, while the Bureau of Health Manpower may provide funds for
expanded training programs in clinical pharmacy and clinical pharmacology.

Substantial progress has also been made in dealing with the complex
problems of drug quality, chemical equivalents, bioavailability, and
clinical equivalency. The Task Force and its staff spent a great deal of
time on these problems. After a thorough review, the Task Force concluded that the lack of clinical equivalency among chemical equivalents
meeting all official standards has been "grossly exaggerated as a major
hazard to the public health."[5] This observation and the recommendation for additional studies hardly settled the issue, but the Task Force
did help to place the discussion on a sounder scientific basis.

A number of studies have been done since then and a limited number of drugs where bioequivalency problems exist have been identified. Further work is in progress. The fact remains, as it did in 1969
when the Task Force reported, that the same amounts of chemically
identical active ingredients, in the same dosage forms, meeting all
official compendial standards, will be bioequivalent with few exceptions. The FDA is competent to deal with these exceptions.

It has now been more than seven years since the Task Force on
Prescription Drugs submitted its final report to the Secretary of HEW.
Many thought that the final report would simply be buried or ignored

by Secretary Finch and a new Republican Administration in February 1969. Quite the opposite was the case. Secretary Finch convened a special advisory panel, chaired by Professor John Dunlop of Harvard, to review the findings and recommendations. With some exceptions, the review panel generally agreed with the findings and recommendations. Congress, particularly the Monopoly Subcommittee of the Small Business Committee, has continued to maintain an active interest in the problems identified by the Task Force. The Senate Finance Committee, and more recently the House of Representatives Ways and Means Committee, have considered the problems of prescription drug coverage for the elderly and drug coverage under national health insurance. In the past few years, the Health Subcommittees in both the Senate and the House have begun to consider a number of these problems as well.

The report also attracted a great deal of interest in academic, industrial, and professional circles. This reflects the importance of the issues and the concern that all involved have in resolving some of the complex problems considered by the Task Force.

There are a number of reasons for the Task Force's ability to make a substantial contribution to identifying and resolving some key policy problems. First, an extraordinary staff under the direction of Dr. Milton Silverman was able to gather, organize, and analyze a wealth of information on drug users, prescribers and dispensers, as well as information on the drug industry and drug insurance. This material was presented in a form that could be examined critically by all concerned. Second, the Task Force had strong support from both Secretary Gardner and Secretary Cohen, and its report was given a fair review by Secretary Finch. Finally, it had a full measure of cooperation not only from the Federal agencies concerned, but also from the host of professional and trade associations, industry representatives, and academic and other consultants who worked with the Task Force. Without this cooperation, little would have been accomplished.

Although a number of issues were clarified by the Task Force and actions were initiated that have resolved many problems that were so vexing a decade ago, new and even more difficult problems, such as adverse drug reactions, poor patient adherence to therapeutic regimens, and the rising cost of drug development and testing, have come to the fore. These issues need to be attacked with the same vigor, objectivity and spirit of cooperation that characterized the work of the Task Force on Prescription Drugs.

REFERENCES

1. Task Force on Prescription Drugs, Final Report. Washington, D.C., Department of Health, Education and Welfare, 1969, p. 86.

2. *Op. cit.*; p. 30.

3. Task Force on Prescription Drugs, Interim Report and Recommendations. Washington, D.C., Department of Health, Education and Welfare, 1968, p. 4.

4. *Op. cit.*, ref. 1. p. xii.

5. *Op. cit.*, ref. 1. p. XIX.

Editor's Note

As noted in Dr. Lee's paper, a Review Committee was appointed to review the findings and recommendations of the Task Force on Prescription Drugs. The report of the Review Committee is reproduced here in its entirety.

As noted in the submission letter, only one member of the committee dissented. An excerpt from that dissenting opinion, by Joseph F. Follmann, follows.

[Haworth co-indexing entry note]: "Editor's Note." Smith, Mickey C. Co-published simultaneously in *Journal of Research in Pharmaceutical Economics* (Pharmaceutical Products Press, an imprint of The Haworth Press, Inc.) Vol. 10, No. 4, 2001, p. 193; and: *Prescription Drugs Under Medicare: The Legacy of the Task Force on Prescription Drugs* (ed: Mickey C. Smith) Pharmaceutical Products Press, an imprint of The Haworth Press, Inc., 2001, p. 193. Single or multiple copies of this article are available for a fee from The Haworth Document Delivery Service [1-800-342-9678, 9:00 a.m. - 5:00 p.m. (EST). E-mail address: getinfo@haworthpressinc.com].

Report of the Secretary's Review Committee of the Task Force on Prescription Drugs

Office of the Secretary
U.S. DEPARTMENT OF
HEALTH, EDUCATION, AND WELFARE
Washington, D.C.

HARVARD UNIVERSITY

JOHN T. DUNLOP
David A. Wells
Professor of Political Economy

1737 CAMBRIDGE STREET, G-4
CAMBRIDGE, MASSACHUSETTS 02138

July 23, 1969

Honorable Robert H. Finch
Secretary of Health, Education,
    and Welfare
Washington, D.C.

Dear Secretary Finch:

On March 24, 1969 you appointed a Committee to Review the Findings and Recommendations of the Department's Task Force on Prescription Drugs. The Committee members, from outside government,

[Haworth co-indexing entry note]: "Report of the Secretary's Review Committee of the Task Force on Prescription Drugs." Secretary's Review Committee of the Task Force on Prescription Drugs. Co-published simultaneously in *Journal of Research in Pharmaceutical Economics* (Pharmaceutical Products Press, an imprint of The Haworth Press, Inc.) Vol. 10, No. 4, 2001, pp. 195-205; and: *Prescription Drugs Under Medicare: The Legacy of the Task Force on Prescription Drugs* (ed: Mickey C. Smith) Pharmaceutical Products Press, an imprint of The Haworth Press, Inc., 2001, pp. 195-205. Single or multiple copies of this article are available for a fee from The Haworth Document Delivery Service [1-800-342-9678, 9:00 a.m. - 5:00 p.m. (EST). E-mail address: getinfo@haworthpressinc.com].

were drawn from a wide variety of backgrounds and groups. (The list of members of the Review Committee is attached.)

The Report of the Review Committee is attached. As an appendix to the report the individual views of the members of the Review Committee are attached on the four major groups of issues which the Review Committee elected to study.

Very truly yours,

/signed/

John T. Dunlop

JTD/jp
Enclosures
cc: Dr. Roger O. Egeberg

Members of the Review Committee
of the Task Force on Prescription Drugs

John T. Dunlop, Ph.D., *Chairman*
Professor of Political Economy
Harvard University
1737 Cambridge Street, G-4
Cambridge, Massachusetts 02138
Phone: 617-868-7600

Morris Aarons
General Counsel
and Executive Secretary
National Association of
Pharmaceutical Manufacturers
101 Park Avenue
New York, New York 10017
Phone: 212-MU3-1700

John Adriani, M.D.
Chairman, Council on Drugs
American Medical Association
Charity Hospital

1532 Tulane Avenue
New Orleans, Louisiana 70140
Phone: 504-523-2311

William S. Apple, Ph.D.
Executive Director
American Pharmaceutical
Association
2215 Constitution Avenue, N.W.
Washington, D.C. 20037
Phone: 628-4410

Leighton E. Cluff, M.D.
Professor and Chairman
Department of Medicine
University of Florida College of
Medicine
Gainesville, Florida 32601
Phone: 904-392-2881

Marian Wright Edelman
Attorney at Law
1823 Jefferson Place, N.W.
Washington, D.C. 20036
Phone: 659-4240

J. F. Follmann, Jr.
Director of Information &
Research
Health Insurance Association
of America
750 Third Avenue
New York, New York
Phone: 212-YU6-8866

Victor R. Fuchs, Ph.D.
Vice President-Research
National Bureau of Economic
Research
261 Madison Avenue
New York, New York 10016
Phone: 212-682-3190

Thomas H. Hayes, M.D., Ph.D.
Director, Department of Drugs
American Medical Association
535 N. Dearborn Street
Chicago, Illinois 60610
Phone: 312-527-1500

William Hutton
Executive Director
National Council of Senior
Citizens
1627 K Street, N.W.
Washington, D.C. 20006
Phone: 783-6850

George James, M.D.
Dean
Mount Sinai School of Medicine

100th Street & Fifth Avenue
New York, New York 10029
Phone: 212-876-1000, ext. 8654

V. D. Mattia, M.D.
President
Hoffman-LaRoche, Inc.
Nutley, New Jersey 07110
Phone: 201-235-2011

Margaret M. McCarron, M.D.
Assistant Medical Director
Los Angeles County
University of Southern California
Medical Center
Room 1110
1200 N. State Street
Los Angeles, California 90033

Bert Seidman
Director, Department of Society
Security
American Federation of Labor–
Council of Industrial
Organizations
815 Sixteenth Street, N.W.
Washington, D.C. 20006
Phone: NA8-3870

Willard B. Simmons
Executive Secretary
National Association of Retail
Druggists
One East Wacker Drive
Chicago, Illinois 60601
Phone: 312-321-1146

C. Joseph Stetler
President
Pharmaceutical Manufacturers
Association
1155 Fifteenth Street, N.W.
Washington, D.C. 20005
Phone: 296-2440

Warren E. Weaver, Ph.D.
Dean
School of Pharmacy
Medical College of Virginia
Richmond, Virginia 23219
Phone: 703-770-4648

July 22, 1969

Report of the Secretary' Review
Committee of the Task Force on
Prescription Drugs

On March 24, 1969 Secretary of Health, Education and Welfare Robert H. Finch named a 17 member committee to review the findings of the Department's Task Force on Prescription Drugs (Final Report dated February 7, 1969). The committee members, all from outside government, were drawn from a wide variety of backgrounds and groups.

The Task Force on Prescription Drugs was established in May 1967 to undertake a comprehensive study of the problems of including the costs of out-of-hospital prescription drugs under Medicare. The Task Force, under the chairmanship of Dr. Philip R. Lee, Assistant Secretary for Health and Scientific Affairs, made a number of significant studies, issued a series of 10 interim reports and background papers.

This Review Committee was not established to provide a comprehensive evaluation of so extensive a series of reports and technical studies. Nor would this committee be entirely appropriate for an exhaustive review, particularly in a short period and without staff. The assignment of this Review Committee is very much more limited and specialized. Secretary Finch charged the committee as follows: "What I now want, to assist me in determining the course of action I am to take, is the judgment of groups outside government who are directly and vitally concerned with the place of prescription drugs in health care–the medical and pharmacy professions, industry, economics, and the consumers of health services, that is the American people."

At its first meeting on April 4, 1969 this Review Committee decided that it could most effectively fulfill this limited assignment in a brief period by concentrating upon four groups of issues raised in the findings and recommendations of the Task Force.

I. The question of the inclusion of out-of-hospital prescription drugs in Medicare and the major features of any such program.
II. Certain pharmacological issues particularly relating to chemical, biological and clinical equivalency and to federal regulation.
III. Certain economic characteristics of drug manufacturing and drug distribution particularly relating to research, product differentiation and pricing.
IV. The means of improving the flow of information regarding drugs to practicing physicians.

Individual members of this Review Committee then were invited to state their views on each of these four groups of issues. These memoranda prepared by all members of the committee, except the chairman, are attached as an appendix to this report. This appendix is an integral part of the report. It is thus readily possible to ascertain in some detail the shades of views and advice of the diverse groups represented on this Review Committee.

This procedure has simplified the writing of this brief Report since the opinions and arguments of individual members are readily available and stated in their own terms. The brief text of this Report was developed after a discussion of the issues and the memoranda prepared by the individual members at the second meeting held on May 6, 1969. This discussion sought to identify major points of difference, to clarify misunderstandings and to achieve genuine agreement on some questions. The draft text of this Report was thereafter circulated to all members of the Review Committee before its submission and most members suggested specific comments. The chairman bears final responsibility for its formulation.

This Report has sought to indicate areas of general agreement on the four groups of issues and also points of significant difference where they remained. No attempt has been made to achieve artificial agreement. The remaining differences may often be as significant as the area of agreement. This approach is in accordance with Secretary Finch's request: "Let me say further that I do not seek a unanimous report nor any artificial compromise. I would, of course, like to know the points on which you are in complete agreement, but it is equally important for me to know where you differ and why."

I. Out-of-Hospital Prescription Drugs and Medicare

One of the most significant findings of the Task Force on Prescription Drugs provided: "In order to improve the access of the elderly to high quality health care, and to protect them where possible against high drug expenses which they may be unable to meet, there is need for an out-of-hospital drug insurance program under Medicare," (Finding No. 2). It further concluded that such a program would be both economically and medically feasible and should be instituted.

1. This Review Committee concludes, with only one dissent, that the Secretary of Health, Education, and Welfare should recommend an Administration decision for an out-of-hospital drug insurance program under Medicare.

The arguments which seem particularly cogent in support of this conclusion of the committee are as follows: "The requirements for appropriate prescription drug therapy by the elderly are very great–far greater, in fact, than those of any other group–and many elderly men and women are now unable to meet those needs with their limited incomes, savings, or present insurance coverage." (Finding No. 1). Some unnecessary high cost hospital use could be reduced by the provision for out-of-hospital prescription drugs. The present inequity under Medicare between payment for in-hospital drug costs and the absence of any payments for identical out-of-hospital drug usage should be eliminated. Other advanced industrial countries have developed programs for out-of-hospital drug costs under social insurance.

2. The Review Committee recommends overwhelmingly that the Secretary authorize and direct the Commissioner, Social Security Administration in cooperation with other officers of the Department of Health, Education, and Welfare to develop more detailed plans, proposed regulations, data processing procedures and cost computations than presently available in keeping with the major features of a program outlined below, including some alternative variations. Such further details are essential for legislative consideration.

The Task Force appropriately found (Final Report, p. 44) that "considerable time would be required to develop all the necessary administrative mechanisms" and that full implementation of a program would require a substantial period after enactment of appropriate legislation. A decision to proceed with more detailed administrative planning and legislative proposals is necessary if a program is to be operative in two years or so.

3. The Task Force proposed, or suggested that consideration be given, to a variety of features in the design of an insurance program in order to constrain costs. It suggested that initially coverage should be given to prescription drugs most likely to be essential in the treatment of chronic rather than acute disease, that consideration be given to an annual deductible of $50 or $100, or that benefits might be initially restricted to those over some age such as 70 or 72, that a formulary be used in part for the purpose of constricting costs and that utilization review procedures be developed for the same purpose. (Findings No. 31, 32, 33, 18, 28). Some of these proposals such as that relating to a formulary, were advanced in part also for reasons of "high quality medical care" and "rational prescribing."

This Review Committee is well aware that costs of Medicare have greatly exceeded expectations and that the failure to design into a program effective cost constraints may well jeopardize legislative approval of any out-of-hospital prescription drug program. Nonetheless, this committee has reservations concerning a number of these Task Force suggestions. This committee has sought to develop alternative suggestions for cost control, but it recognizes the need for further work in this area with more precise cost estimates as legislative proposals and regulations are developed. It is also aware of the possibilities of increased utilization of prescription drugs, some of which may be unwarranted.

 a. This Review Committee does not regard the limitation to chronic disease treatments and the exclusion of acute cases as advisable or administrable.

 b. An age limitation other than over 65 is undesirable.

 c. An annual deductible provision which imposes a requirement on the patient as an individual to keep records should be avoided.

 d. Co-insurance provisions are less desirable than co-payment features.

e. While value of formularies has been well established for hospitals, most members of the committee are of the view that a required national formulary is not appropriate for an out-of-hospital prescription drug insurance program. A purely advisory national formulary, with utilization review on the basis of the experience of a number of formularies developed on a locality basis, might possibly be appropriate.

4. The Review Committee would favor an out-of-hospital prescription drug program under Medicare which incorporated the following features:

a. A co-payment arrangement so that the patient would be required to pay a fixed dollar amount for each prescription. (It might be possible to incorporate into such a plan an arrangement so that the co-payment would cease, or be reduced, or be subject to reimbursement over a certain accumulated amount during a year.)
b. A vendor reimbursement arrangement so that pharmacists and other vendors rather than beneficiaries would be reimbursed. The committee generally favors a dollar and cents, rather than a percentage, mark up or fee based upon practice in the locality by type of outlet to be added to the acquisition cost of the drug product.
c. Most of the members of the Committee favored a program under Part A of Medicare.
d. Utilization review is essential but costs are difficult to control even with post audit.

5. The Review Committee has made no attempt to compare the relative benefits of an out-of-hospital prescription drug program under Medicare with the benefits of other possible medical programs or other possible alternative expenditures of public funds.

II. Pharmacological Issues

There was general agreement that the establishment of biologic or therapeutic equivalency for generic drug products would result in decreased drug costs for the consumer. Minor variations between different products of the same drugs with low potent pharmacologic action are of less concern, but biologic or therapeutic equivalency in this group of drug products could also result in some reduction of costs for consumers.

The Committee recommends:

1. The Food and Drug Administration continue to develop Reference Standards for generic drugs to assure biologic equivalency among drug products.
2. The Secretary of the Department of Health, Education, and Welfare be assisted by appropriate Advisory Committees to evaluate drug costs and biologic and therapeutic equivalency.

The Committee supports the Task Force Report on the need for effective regulation of quality control in manufacturing of drugs through improved regulations related to the registration or licensing of manufacturers.

III. Economic Features of Drug Manufacturing and Drug Distribution

1. Drug industry research. There seems to be general agreement that the Task Force finding concerning duplicative and wasteful research by drug manufacturers was not adequately documented in the Task Force Report. Beyond that, some members of the Review Committee believe that the finding could not be documented because it is essentially incorrect. Others are prepared to give more credence to the charge while still others suggest that it might have been true in the 1950's and early 1960's, but is not true of current drug industry research.

2. Drug industry profits. There is general agreement that drug industry profits have been and are high compared with other industries, and that this situation requires careful study to determine its causes and implications.

3. Physician-owned repackaging companies. There is general agreement with the finding that products marketed by physician-owned repackaging companies should be considered unacceptable for reimbursement except in those instances in which the Secretary of

Health, Education, and Welfare determines that the availability of products marketed by such companies is in the public interest.

4. Pharmacy research. There is general agreement with the recommendation that the National Center for Health Services Research and Development should develop and support research to improve the efficiency and effectiveness of community and hospital pharmacy operations.

5. Price differences. The subject was not discussed at the committee meeting, but in the written statements of committee members there is broad support for the recommendation of a study to consider the substantial differences in the prices at which drug products are offered to community pharmacies and to hospitals and government agencies.

6. Price information. This subject was not discussed by the committee, but in the written statements there is broad support for the finding of a need for medical associations, pharmacy associations, and consumer groups to develop, at the local level, mechanisms whereby patients may obtain information on local prescription prices.

IV. Information and Identification

The Committee addressed itself most particularly to the flow of information on drugs to physicians. Most of the Committee generally concurred with the Task Force recommendation No. 10 regarding a publication providing up-to-date information and guidelines on drug therapy. Most felt that the Department of Health, Education, and Welfare should support this effort which should preferably be the work of non-government drug experts. In general the Committee concurred with recommendation No. 12, regarding a compendium, except that there is not uniformity on the question of authorship. Those members expressing an opinion in the majority favored an authoritative compendium which would be supported by government but published by a non-government authority. It might be useful to pre-test any compendium.

Recommendations concerned with continuing education of physicians and courses in clinical pharmacology in medical schools all relate to the potential long range effects of kinds of information that affect the prescribing habits of physicians. Time did not permit full and complete discussion of these issues but those commenting favor a constructive approach to these problems. In a similar way, recommendations relating to education of pharmacists and pharmacist aides evoke a response indicating that need for pharmacist aides is not clearly demonstrated at this time and should await a more definitive study of the role of the pharmacist in the dissemination of drug information and in drug distribution. Those commenting favor a study that would bring the dimensions of the problem into clearer focus, as recommended in part by the Task Force.

Secretary's Review Committee
of the Task Force on Prescription Drugs:
Dissenting Comments

Joseph F. Follmann

The Committee has been appointed to review the Findings and Recommendations of the Department of HEW's Task Force on Prescription Drugs. It has not been asked to develop, initiate, or recommend a program of its own.

The Report of the Task Force is not a simple matter to address oneself to. The body of the Report is a mixture of fact findings, which may or may not be correct; several unsubstantiated speculations; and a body of material of questionable relevance to the subject or purposes of the Report. At the same time, it leaves undiscussed and unanswered some matters of direct pertinence and importance to the subject. The Report then documents its Findings. These are not a statement of factual findings by the Task Force, but include surmise, material of questionable relevance, and conclusions which appear to be much more in the nature of recommendations arrived at after trying to compromise such difficult matters as benefits, costs, sources of financing, and administration. Yet, when one examines the Recommendations, and despite the Findings, no program whatever is recommended with respect to adding a prescription drug benefit to the Medicare program; and consequently there are no Recommendations with respect to what such an addition would constitute in the way of benefits, costs, financing, and administration. Instead, the Recommendations are concerned with matters which appear for the most part irrelevant, particularly since no program is recommended.

[Haworth co-indexing entry note]: "Secretary's Review Committee of the Task Force on Prescription Drugs: Dissenting Comments." Follmann, Joseph F. Co-published simultaneously in *Journal of Research in Pharmaceutical Economics* (Pharmaceutical Products Press, an imprint of The Haworth Press, Inc.) Vol. 10, No. 4, 2001, pp. 207-209; and: *Prescription Drugs Under Medicare: The Legacy of the Task Force on Prescription Drugs* (ed: Mickey C. Smith) Pharmaceutical Products Press, an imprint of The Haworth Press, Inc., 2001, pp. 207-209. Single or multiple copies of this article are available for a fee from The Haworth Document Delivery Service [1-800-342-9678, 9:00 a.m. - 5:00 p.m. (EST). E-mail address: getinfo@haworth pressinc.com].

Since neither the Report nor the Findings make a clear case for adding such a benefit to the Medicare program, despite the fact that Finding No. 2 says there is a "need," it seems sufficient to express concurrence with the fact that no program is recommended. This would seem particularly advisable at this time since the cost of the Medicare program is at present unsettled and should be resolved before any additions are made to the program.

There are members of the Committee, however, who will not concur in this conclusion. Therefore, some discussion of certain details of the Report is necessary, based upon the outlined [sic] agreed upon at the April 4, 1969 meeting of the Committee.

I. AN INSURED PLAN

1. Should the Secretary Recommend an Insured Plan?

No. The Task Force Report has not made a case for, nor has it recommended, the addition of an out-of-hospital prescription drug program to the Medicare program. The facts stated in the Findings show that 51% of the aged have supplemental private health insurance benefits. While it is stated that only 9% have private health insurance coverage for drugs, this can be misleading, since any type of supplemental benefit relieves individual funds which can then be used for the purchase of drugs. The Report recognizes that an additional role can be played by Medicaid, but does not attempt to show what role Medicaid actually plays or could play in the payment of drugs for Medicare beneficiaries. The Report recognizes that such matters as tax relief, other public assistance programs, and OEO clinics all can play a role with respect to payment for drugs, but does not delineate this role. Beyond this, it appears that some 12 to 15% of the aged incur prescribed drug bills in excess of $100, and about 9% receive drugs with no cost to the patient. Such facts are only glimmers of the situation as respects older people. What is needed is data which relate the ability of older people who are heavy users of drugs to pay for such drugs, as well as the number of the aged who have financial problems with respect to the cost of drugs, after taking full cognizance of the role of Medicaid and other means of assistance available to the aged since it would indicate the type of program, if any, which would be needed. This is necessary before any decision could be made with respect to the inclusion of drugs in Medicare.

Incidentally, the discussion of drugs in Government programs in other nations dismisses without much notice the difficulties which these programs have occasioned. Finding No. 10, for example, says that these programs are shown to be "economically feasible." This statement seems to be subject to considerable doubt. There is evidence that these programs have run into considerable problems and this should be examined more carefully before a decision would be made. The Report, for example, does not go on to say that in the United Kingdom charges for drugs had to be reinstituted by the Labour Government.

End of Excerpt

Editor's Note

As stated in the introduction, we cannot give this Congressional performance its due. Surely it is a bizarre example of the American political process at work. We refer to the "Catastrophic" Drug Bill here primarily because the legislation which put Medicare prescription medication coverage into place (P. L. 100-360) did not have the benefit of the kind of study provided by the Task Force. Confusion, conflicting estimates as to the ultimate costs, disagreement concerning the technology necessary to provide immediate drug utilization review, political maneuvering by virtually every group with an interest–all resulted in what, one hopes, was the embarrassing *repeal* of the act. Ironically, the vote to repeal in the House of Representatives (360-66) exceeded the 328-72 House vote that adopted the legislation the year before.

But that's another worthwhile, but too long for here, story.

John Iglehart's report in the *New England Journal of Medicine* was published not long before the repeal. In that context, we believe it belongs in this collection.

[Haworth co-indexing entry note]: "Editor's Note." Smith, Mickey C. Co-published simultaneously in *Journal of Research in Pharmaceutical Economics* (Pharmaceutical Products Press, an imprint of The Haworth Press, Inc.) Vol. 10, No. 4, 2001, p. 211; and: *Prescription Drugs Under Medicare: The Legacy of the Task Force on Prescription Drugs* (ed: Mickey C. Smith) Pharmaceutical Products Press, an imprint of The Haworth Press, Inc., 2001, p. 211. Single or multiple copies of this article are available for a fee from The Haworth Document Delivery Service [1-800-342-9678, 9:00 a.m. - 5:00 p.m. (EST). E-mail address: getinfo@haworthpressinc.com].

Health Policy Report:
Medicare's New Benefits:
"Catastrophic" Health Insurance

John K. Iglehart

Medicare's new health insurance benefit for catastrophic illness, proposed by the Reagan administration and expanded by a Congress hungry to demonstrate its election-year fealty to the elderly, nevertheless incorporates an important policy that is consistent with the government's budget woes: the elderly will pay for the benefit themselves through larger premiums based mostly on their individual financial circumstances. The expansion also reflects another reality–that the growth of federal spending on health may have moderated during the Reagan presidency, but it still outstripped every other major programmatic area with the exception of interest on the national debt. As a result, government's involvement in medical care is more formidable than ever before.

Reagan, declaring the catastrophic-illness benefit an important extension of the financial protection for the nation's elderly, signed the Medicare Catastrophic Coverage Act of 1988 (P.L. 100-360) into law on July 1. The President's action capped a convoluted saga that began officially 30 months earlier with his 1986 State of the Union address, in which he directed the Department of Health and Human Services to develop options in collaboration with the private sector that could lead to better protection for all Americans against the economic consequences of serious illness. The recipient of Reagan's directive was Health and

---

Reprinted with permission from the *New England Journal of Medicine* 1989; 320: 329-35. Copyright © 1989 Massachusetts Medical Society. All rights reserved.

[Haworth co-indexing entry note]: "Health Policy Report: Medicare's New Benefits: 'Catastrophic' Health Insurance." Iglehart, John K. Co-published simultaneously in *Journal of Research in Pharmaceutical Economics* (Pharmaceutical Products Press, an imprint of The Haworth Press, Inc.) Vol. 10, No. 4, 2001, pp. 213-228; and: *Prescription Drugs Under Medicare: The Legacy of the Task Force on Prescription Drugs* (ed: Mickey C. Smith) Pharmaceutical Products Press, an imprint of The Haworth Press, Inc., 2001, pp. 213-228.

Human Services Secretary Otis R. Bowen, a former Indiana governor and family practitioner who had already declared at his nomination hearing in December 1985 that the enactment of a Medicare catastrophic-illness benefit would be one of his "main priorities" as secretary.

During the period before Reagan's pronouncement directing Bowen to study the issue and right up to the day the measure became law, some of the President's more conservative loyalists, the commercial health insurance industry, and the pharmaceutical lobby sought unsuccessfully to kill the initiative. Opponents of a Medicare catastrophic-illness benefit within the administration viewed the program expansion as inconsistent with Reagan's commitment to restrain federal spending for social programs and to use private-sector solutions whenever possible. The elements of the commercial-insurance industry that opposed it, particularly Mutual of Omaha, viewed the legislation as a threat to their "medigap" insurance business, which provides coverage for expenses not covered by Medicare. In contrast, the Blue Cross and Blue Shield Association supported the legislation. The seemingly endless maneuvering that took place in the crafting of this law was testimony to how complex the public policy process has become and how politically attractive the expansion of federal social service programs remains–even for a Ronald Reagan, under the right circumstances–despite all the arguments to the contrary.

Throughout the process, Congress never directly addressed some of the more fundamental questions of resource allocation that arose in relation to the concentration of more medical spending for high-technology care on the segment of the population that is already the most heavily insured. Small steps were taken to provide financial protection to a fraction of the approximately 37 million Americans who lack health insurance. Congress also demonstrated a new sensitivity to the issue of not passing along the cost of the new benefit to the next generation or tapping general revenues to pay for it. Senator Lloyd M. Bentsen (D-Tex.), chairman of the Senate Finance Committee and a cosponsor of the legislation, addressed this issue last June 8 during the floor debate:

> I remind my colleagues that these benefit improvements will not cost the Treasury one dollar. This is not a bill that passes the costs on to the younger generation. The premiums will be paid by

those people who are 65 years or older and who today are doing better financially than any other age group.

In this report, I will discuss the new benefit program and how it will be financed. I also will report on the political dimensions of the debate in terms of a struggle between the Reagan administration, which captured the political high ground by proposing it in the first place, and the Democratic legislators (particularly Representatives John D. Dingell of Michigan, Dan Rostenkowski of Illinois, Fortney H. [Pete] Stark and Henry A. Waxman, both of California, and Senators Bentsen, Thomas A. Daschle of South Dakota, and George J. Mitchell of Maine) who demonstrated their fidelity to the elderly by expanding the plan substantially. Bowen and his chief of staff, Thomas R. Burke, and Representative Willis D. Gradison, Jr., (Ohio) and Senators John H. Chafee (R.I.), Robert J. Dole (Kans.), David F. Durenberger (Minn.), and H. John Heinz III (Pa.) also had important roles on the Republican side. The private interests that lobby on behalf of the elderly–the insurance industry, pharmaceutical manufacturers, and other concerns–were important elements of the equation, too. Though they were supportive, the providers of medical care, as represented by the American Medical Association, the American Hospital Association, and other like-minded advocates, did not become centrally involved because they viewed the legislation as a matter involving beneficiaries. However, their constituencies stand to gain from the estimated \$30.8 billion in new Medicare outlays that will flow to providers on behalf of beneficiaries as a consequence of the law in the period from 1989 to 1993.

The federal action represents the most sweeping expansion of Medicare benefits since the program's creation in 1965. Over the next three years, when the benefits will be phased in, Medicare will place a cap on patients' obligation to share the costs of hospital coverage. It will limit, but not absolutely cap, beneficiary payments for Part B physicians' and related services (because nonparticipating doctors and medical suppliers can still bill for more than Medicare's approved charge). In addition, it will pay for all allowable outpatient prescription-drug charges after a deductible has been reached and a copayment covered. Finally, it will provide some elements of a benefit for long-term care–expansion in coverage for care at home, in a hospice, and in a skilled-nursing facility.

Under the law, beneficiaries who reach the financial thresholds that trigger catastrophic-illness coverage must do so by incurring expenses for cost-sharing (i.e., deductibles and copayments) that result directly from their use of Medicare benefits. When all the ceilings on spending by beneficiaries take effect in 1991, there will be three parts: a $560 cap on inpatient hospital services, a limit of $1,370 on physicians' and other Part B services, and a limit of $600 on costs incurred for outpatient drugs. Beneficiaries will still be required to pay 50 percent coinsurance for drug expenditures above that ceiling. The administration proposed only a single overall cap of $2,000 for hospital and physicians' expenses, but Congress decided on separate ceilings because the program itself is divided between Parts A and B, and the jurisdiction of the congressional committee over Medicare is split likewise.

Even with the enactment of the new benefit, a substantial percentage of an average elderly person's health care bill would not be covered by Medicare, including such items as long-term care, dental services, eyeglasses, and most preventive services. Calling the program expansion a catastrophic-illness benefit may be appropriate in the case of some beneficiaries whose afflictions are covered, but the measure falls short of dealing with every contingency. The most conspicuous omission is coverage for long-term care, which costs an average of $25,000 a year for people who need it. The Congressional Budget Office estimates that once the new act is fully effective, about 22 percent of enrollees will be entitled to higher payments for Medicare benefits because of the hospital insurance provisions, the Part B cap, or the new drug coverage.[1] The House Ways and Means Committee, in estimates distributed December 6, said some 7.8 million Medicare beneficiaries will receive new Medicare benefits each year when the law is fully implemented: 1.5 million will be spared the obligation to pay more than one hospital deductible a year, 2.4 million will have Part B copayments in excess of the catastrophic illness cap, and 5.8 million will receive prescription-drug benefits. In addition, states will be required to cover the cost-sharing expenses of 2.7 million poor people who could not otherwise afford to participate in Medicare.

EXPANDED COVERAGE FOR SHORT-TERM CARE

The law provides unlimited coverage for short-term hospital care, effective January 1989, to Medicare's 32 million elderly and disabled beneficiaries, after the fulfillment of one annual deductible ($560). Previously, Medicare payment for inpatient stays ceased after beneficiaries had used 90 days during a "spell of illness" and had exhausted their lifetime reserve of 60 days. To obtain this coverage, inpatients (or their medigap insurance policies, which about 62 percent of eligible beneficiaries purchase) were required to pay a deductible ($540 in 1988) for every spell of illness. In addition, patients paid daily coinsurance charges equal to one quarter of the inpatient hospital deductible for days 61 to 90 during a spell of illness ($135 in 1988) and an even higher daily coinsurance charge for the remaining 60 lifetime reserve days ($270 a day in 1988). Striking a blow for simplicity, but also to provide catastrophic-illness coverage, Congress repealed these cost-sharing requirements and the concepts of a spell of illness and reserve days in favor of the single annual hospital deductible.

Once the annual deductible has been paid, Medicare will provide benefits for all inpatient care that is covered, regardless of the amount, the length of stay, or the number of times admitted in any one year. (The current 190-day lifetime limit on inpatient services in a psychiatric hospital remains unchanged.) A hospital's ability to take advantage of this broadened coverage for purposes of reimbursement will be held in check by Medicare's prospective payment system, which pays fixed amounts based on the determination of diagnosis-related group (DRG). Most cases of catastrophic illness involve several DRG categories and become so-called outliers; the amount of payment for such cases is based on established formulas.

During the several years that passed while Congress considered the legislation, the members became far more aware that Medicare finances short-term, not long-term care. Despite efforts by Representative Claude D. Pepper (D-Fla.) to expand Medicare to include more coverage for long-term care, an issue Congress is certain to revisit, Medicare remains designed essentially to assist only acutely ill patients. Nevertheless, Congress did recognize the need to remove the longstanding, artificial distinction in the continuum of care by eliminating, effective 1989, the requirement that patients must be in a hospital for at least three consecutive days before being admitted to a skilled-nursing facility. In addition, the number of days for which a beneficiary is eligible for skilled nursing care was changed from 100 per benefit period to 150 days per year. The cost-sharing arrangements were also restructured to provide better protection against catastrophic costs. There is no deductible for skilled nursing care. For the first eight days of care, however, the patient pays 20 percent of the national average daily rate for care in a skilled-nursing facility–an estimated $25.50 per day in 1989. After that, there is no additional cost. Effective 1989, after 210 days of care in a hospice, beneficiaries will be eligible for unlimited hospice care if they are recertified as still being terminally ill by a medical director of the facility or an attending physician.

The law also liberalizes Medicare's benefit for home health care. Effective January 1990, home health services for patients will be expanded to a maximum of 38 consecutive days of daily care if they meet the same restrictive eligibility requirements that applied previously–the beneficiary must be homebound, need skilled rather than custodial care, or need physical or speech therapy. This limit can be extended if deemed medically appropriate. There are no limits to coverage for intermittent care. The interpretation made by the Health Care Financing Administration (HCFA) of the requirement that home health care be intermittent, which was under court challenge at the time, limited the frequency of daily visits to no more than five days a week for up to three consecutive weeks. Previously, no limit was placed on the overall number of intermittent visits, and there was no coinsurance requirement for home health visits. Under the new law these provisions did not change.

PHYSICIANS' SERVICES

An important feature of the new law is the limit imposed on expenses incurred for services covered under Medicare's Part B–principally charges for physicians' services, but also those of outpatient clinics, clinical laboratory charges, and fees for hospital outpatient services, effective January 1990. Currently, there is no such limit. Under the new law, after a beneficiary has incurred expenses of $1,370 in 1990 for Part B services, Medicare will pay 100 percent of the reasonable charge of any additional Part B service. The ceiling was indexed for future years (to reach an estimated $1,900 by 1993) as a cost-constraining device, so that a constant share of beneficiaries (7 percent) will exceed it and use Part B catastrophic-illness benefits every year. Only expenses for cost sharing that is related to Medicare-approved charges count toward the Part B out-of-pocket limit. When a beneficiary is billed for a physician's services at rates higher than Medicare's approved rates under so-called balance billing, the additional amount is not applicable to the ceiling. Representative Brian Donnelly (D-Mass.) sought to incorporate a provision into the new legislation that barred balance billing, but it was never seriously considered by Congress.

In the one instance in which the new law recognizes preventive services, Part B will pay for mammography screening of elderly and disabled women on a periodic basis, effective 1990. However, out of concern over the demand that might be created for such coverage and the quality of care that might be rendered by clinics established for this purpose, Congress directed the Physician Payment Review Commission and the General Accounting Office to examine these questions. Currently, the only preventive services covered by Medicare are for vaccines to counter hepatitis B, influenza, and pneumonia.

The other expansion of Part B benefits underscored the growing congressional interest in broadening Medicare beyond its traditional focus–namely, by incorporating a small benefit for long-term care. As of 1990, Medicare will provide a respite benefit for chronically dependent persons who are trying to avoid entering a nursing home but cannot do so without assistance with the essential activities of daily living, such as bathing, eating, and using the toilet. Under this provision, Medicare will pay 80 percent of the reasonable costs of in-home personal services and nursing care for up to 80 hours a year, in order to give the usual caretaker of a homebound patient some relief, or respite. Payments under the respite benefit will be triggered only after a patient has accumulated substantial medical expenses in a given year. Defending the benefit on the House floor last June 2, Representative Waxman, chairman of the House Energy and Commerce Subcommittee on Health and the Environment, said:

> This is a small first step toward dealing with long-term care, but it is strategically the most vital first step. Moreover, it demonstrates that the Medicare program can be used creatively to meet the needs of the Medicare population, without regard to preconceived notions and that the program must be limited to acute care.

PRESCRIPTION-DRUG COVERAGE

The provisions of the catastrophic-illness law that created the most controversy dealt with the decision of Congress to extend Medicare coverage to outpatient prescription drugs for the first time. The administration had not sought this benefit and acquiesced to it only reluctantly. Ironically, most manufacturers of brand-name pharmaceuticals opposed it, too. The American Association of Retired Persons (AARP) and manufacturers of generic drugs supported the legislation, as did the organizations that represent community pharmacies, chain drug stores, and mail-service pharmacies. Currently, Medicare pays only for prescription drugs administered in the hospital or a skilled nursing facility, injections by physicians, and immunosuppressive drugs furnished during the year after an organ transplantation. Beginning in 1990, Medicare will cover immunosuppressive drugs after a transplantation beyond the current one-year limit, subject to a $550 deductible and an initial coinsurance rate of 50 percent. This coverage will be provided whether or not the transplantation was paid for by Medicare. The program will also begin paying for intravenous drugs administered at home, subject to a 20 percent coinsurance payment and a $550 deductible that is waived if the use of such drugs began in the hospital. Beginning in 1991, coverage for all other outpatient prescription drugs, biologic agents, and insulin will be added. Beneficiaries will be required to meet yearly deductibles of $600 in 1991 and $652 in 1992. Coinsurance is set at 50 percent in 1991, 40 percent in 1992, and 20 percent in 1993 and thereafter.

The administration's greatest concern over the outpatient drug benefit is its cost. Estimates by the HCFA and the Congressional Budget Office have varied widely. The HCFA estimated considerably higher outlays for the benefit than did the Congressional Budget Office, but Congress established the premium levels in the statute on the basis of the projections of its budget office. The agencies disagreed over the extent of the demand that the new drug benefit would generate and made widely varying predictions of prescription-drug use in 1991, based on extrapolations from the available data bases. The Congressional Budget Office estimated that 16.8 percent of Medicare beneficiaries would spend beyond the limit of the drug deductible and use the benefit in 1991 and 1992, whereas the HCFA projected that 25 percent of beneficiaries would do so. As a consequence of the HCFA's higher cost estimate, that agency's actuaries now predict a deficit of almost $500 million for 1991 in the Catastrophic Drug Insurance Trust Fund and, if no action is taken, a shortfall of $4.5 billion by 1993. The new legislation directs both agencies to refine their drug estimates in 1989, when more recent survey data become available.

The outpatient drug benefit also proved controversial because of the opposition of the Pharmaceutical Manufacturers Association (PMA). In many instances, the private interests that lobby for providers of care or medical suppliers encourage third-party efforts to expand benefits coverage, although the government cost controls that now usually accompany broader benefits make the results of such activity less certain. In contrast, the PMA, which enlisted outside public relations consultants and lobbyists, waged an aggressive grass-roots campaign to persuade the elderly that coverage of outpatient drugs by Medicare would not serve their interests. Currently, the AARP estimates that elderly people pay for 81 percent of their outpatient prescription drugs out of their own pockets. Many medigap insurance policies do not cover the cost of such drugs.

The PMA, whose 100 manufacturer members produce most of the prescription drugs used in the United States, argued that Medicare coverage of drugs could lead to the creation of a formulary that might limit the availability of some drugs to the elderly and could also prompt the government to impose price controls on drugs to the detriment of the research-intensive industry. There was also concern about provisions in the law that create incentives for pharmacists to dispense generic drugs whenever medically appropriate. Although the PMA's campaign slowed consideration of the legislation and led to an amendment prohibiting the Department of Health and Human Services from establishing a formulary for all beneficiaries (an exception to this ban was made in the case of health maintenance organizations, many of which already have established formularies), its effort to kill the drug benefit failed. The exercise also annoyed many legislators, who took exception to the PMA's campaign because they believed it sought to persuade leaders of the elderly groups to do the industry's bidding when the primary goal of the effort was to maintain the pricing flexibility and profits of the pharmaceutical companies. The AARP also took exception to the PMA's grass-roots campaign, as did several manufacturers, including Merck, Johnson & Johnson, and G. D. Searle.

One of the major long-range consequences of the outpatient drug benefit will be to change the existing relations among physicians, patients, pharmacists, and drug companies. Concerned over the cost and utilization consequences of the new benefit, Congress wrote into the law provisions requiring the Department of Health and Human Services to establish a program that would identify, in the words of the conference report (no. 100-661),

> (i) instances and patterns of unnecessary or inappropriate prescribing or dispensing practices; (ii) instances or patterns of substandard care; and (iii) potential adverse drug reactions. The conferees expect that participating pharmacists will review the medication profile of beneficiaries for potential adverse reactions before filling prescriptions. The conferees further intend that carriers will review claims retrospectively to identify practitioners exhibiting a pattern of inappropriate drug prescribing or dispensing.

The HCFA will provide every participating pharmacy with a communications device or appropriate software through which the pharmacy must transmit to a data bank information about all outpatient prescriptions dispensed for Medicare beneficiaries. The principal purpose of this practice is to ensure the quick determination of a beneficiary's total out-of-pocket payments that are eligible for the annual deductible, in order to ascertain whether the beneficiary is eligible for drug coverage. But such data will also constitute a vast new source of information about patterns in the prescription of outpatient drugs that the HCFA, private third-party payers, the pharmaceutical industry, and individual researchers can use for other purposes, subject to the requirements of patient confidentiality. When the drug benefit is fully implemented in 1991, the HCFA estimates that it will generate 700 million new Medicare claims, more than double the load of claims processed by the program at present.

ASSISTANCE TO LOW-INCOME PERSONS

The new law incorporates several important provisions that will ease the burden of medical expenses for low-income elderly persons. These provisions are a tribute to the tenacity of Representative Waxman, who time and again has advanced his vision of a more expansive role for government in the financing of medical care for the elderly and the impoverished, despite the efforts of the Reagan administration and more faint-hearted Democrats. In this instance, Waxman persuaded Congress to require the states, on a phased basis, to expand Medicaid funds to pay the Medicare premiums, deductibles, and coinsurance for the elderly and disabled who had incomes below the federal poverty level. Sen. Mitchell was instrumental in persuading the Senate to accept this provision. When fully implemented (in 1992), this provision will protect about 2.5 million poor, elderly, and disabled Medicare beneficiaries from the cost-sharing requirements of the catastrophic-illness benefits.

The law addresses another reality of life for the elderly under current Medicaid provisions: that most couples must now impoverish themselves before one member of the pair becomes eligible for nursing home coverage. The new law protects minimal levels of income ($786 a month in 1989) and the assets of a spouse living at home while a husband or wife receives nursing home care financed through Medicaid. The higher-income thresholds to which this provision applies will broaden Medicaid's constituency slightly beyond poor people–a first step, perhaps, in expanding the program to cover more of the nation's uninsured citizens. Finally, the law requires all states, on a phased basis, to extend Medicaid coverage to low-income pregnant women (those with incomes below 100 percent of the poverty level) and their infants by July 1990. Previously, 36 states provided this benefit at their option. The law will extend coverage to an estimated 68,000 poor, pregnant women and 240,000 poor infants by 1990.

The Medicaid provisions that were incorporated in the new law illustrated the creative tension at play in the policy process. Because of the broadening of Medicare coverage, the states with the more generous Medicaid programs would have realized substantial savings in their Medicaid outlays. Representatives Stark and Gradison developed the notion that these savings should be captured for health-related purposes instead of being diverted by the states to other uses. These congressmen were instrumental in imposing new federal requirements on states to use Medicaid dollars to pay the Medicare cost-sharing fees of the poor. Representative Waxman promoted the use of the savings to mandate states to protect against the impoverishment of one spouse as a requirement for the other to receive benefits and to broaden prenatal care benefits for poor women.

BENEFIT FINANCING

Although the drug benefit provoked considerable heat, it may pale in comparison to the surprise that some affluent older people will register when they fill out their income-tax forms for 1989 and learn that the new benefits are mostly financed through a supplemental premium. The Congressional Budget Office estimates that as a consequence of the catastrophic-illness law, new costs for Medicare benefits and administration for fiscal years 1989 through 1993 will total $30.8 billion. With the cost of the new benefits included, total Medicare outlays will reach an estimated $98.5 billion in 1989 and rise to $160 billion by 1993. The Congressional Budget Office calculates that 34 percent of the costs of the new benefits will be for broadened hospital insurance coverage, 50 percent for Part B benefits, and 16 percent for drug coverage.

Initially, the Reagan administration proposed that the new benefits should be financed by the elderly themselves, regardless of financial status, through a monthly increase of $4.92 in the $27.90 premium for Part B coverage, raising the premium to almost $400 annually. Congress agreed with the concept of self-financing, but many legislators and policy analysts viewed the use of the administration's flat premium as the sole revenue source as a regressive measure. Congress did add $4.00 a month to the Part B premium to be paid by every beneficiary in 1989, bringing it to $31.90 a month. But the bulk (63 percent) of the new monies needed to pay for the new benefits will be derived from a mandatory supplemental premium (opponents called it a new tax) paid by approximately 40 percent of eligible beneficiaries on the basis of their income-tax liability. Effective in 1989, each beneficiary will pay $22.50 a year (a 15 percent surtax) as a supplemental premium for every $150 of federal income tax owed. Most will pay the premium along with their income tax. The new law limits the amount of the supplemental premium a beneficiary must pay in 1989 to $800 for an individual and $1,600 for a couple. An estimated 10 percent of enrollees will pay these maximal amounts in 1989, but they represent some of the most articulate members of the elderly, who may be in a position to press their case before the government.[2]

In a front-page article in *The New York Times* November 2 entitled "New Health Insurance Plan Provokes Outcry over Costs," Martin

Tolchin explained the "calculated decision" of Congress to agree to self-financing and an income-related supplemental premium:

> As a group, the elderly have in recent years benefited more than the general population from social programs, and have become more prosperous than the general population. The poverty rate of the elderly declined to 12.4 percent in 1987 from 15.3 percent in 1980, while the poverty rate of the general population increased to 13.6 percent in 1987 from 13 percent in 1980.

Another factor that weighed heavily in the decision of Congress to impose this supplemental premium on the more affluent elderly is that Medicare is subsidized by the population under 65. For example, the current $31.90 monthly Part B premium covers about 25 percent of an enrollee's Part B insurance costs. Virtually all the rest ($32.7 billion in fiscal 1989) is derived from general federal revenues. In addition, the bulk of the annual contribution of $1,838 for Part A insurance is paid by current workers and employers through payroll taxes. The Congressional Budget Office estimates that the total subsidy value of Medicare benefits per enrollee will be $2,024 on average in 1989, and will grow to $3,184 by 1993. The subsidy will be more for low-income enrollees and less for higher-income enrollees who must pay the supplemental premium.

Congress was also prepared to take this step because some 62 percent of the elderly already supplement their Medicare coverage with medigap insurance policies. The law requires that such policies be adjusted to reflect the new changes in Medicare and prohibits insurers from offering duplicate coverage. Congress anticipated that these changes would lower medigap premiums or lower the increases in premium rates, although recent rate increases announced by the AARP, commercial insurers, and Blue Cross and Blue Shield as a consequence of rising medical costs have caused concern in the health policy community. Congress also provided for the establishment of new minimal standards for medigap insurance policies. During the debate, most legislators thought that Medicare expansion represented a better bargain for the elderly than supplemental private policies. (The latest available data, which the General Accounting Office presented to the House Ways and Means Subcommittee on Health on March 10, 1987, showed that in 1985, commercial medigap insurers had a weighted average loss ratio–the percentage of premiums returned to policyholders as benefits–of 65.8 percent. The comparable figure for Blue Cross and Blue Shield plans was 88.6 percent.) On June 2, 1988, Representative Dingell, the chairman of the House Energy and Commerce Committee, expressed a view on the House floor that reflected the majority opinion:

> Over 97 percent of every dollar collected will be returned to beneficiaries, a rate no private insurer could guarantee. . . . This bill will address very specifically the problem of the so-called medigap insurance, duplicative service, and some of the shoddy offerings which are made by some of the less responsible insurance companies.

THE POLITICS OF COVERAGE FOR CATASTROPHIC ILLNESS

Legislation for health insurance for catastrophic illness was hardly a new idea. A variety of proposals had been introduced over the past 15 years by Democrats and Republicans, but none had ever been touted as a presidential priority. What made the latest effort almost a foregone conclusion from the outset was the endorsement of President Reagan–a surprising political twist akin to President Nixon's renewal of American ties to Communist China. As a consequence, once the administration's proposal had been advanced, the central question was not whether Congress would enact the measure, but how. During this process legislators, long stifled in their desire to add an important new benefit to a federal health program, demonstrated an irresistible urge to expand the initial offering.

The bidding began soon after Reagan unveiled his proposal in a variety of private meetings with House Democratic leaders. In the Ways and Means Subcommittee on Health, Representatives Stark and Gradison let it be known early on that Reagan's proposal was a fine starting point. The momentum grew when the AARP declared its reluctance to support a bill for catastrophic-illness insurance that did not expand Medicare coverage in some substantial way, such as adding an outpatient drug benefit. The AARP took its case to House Speaker Jim Wright (D-Tex.), then new to the job and wanting to dispel the notion that he was considerably more conservative than his predecessor, Thomas P. (Tip) O'Neill, Jr. In a key meeting between

Wright and other House Democratic stalwarts, including 88-year-old Claude Pepper, who was then pressing for a wholesale expansion of home health care, and Henry Waxman, who had already drafted language with which a drug benefit could be incorporated, the Speaker declared that he wanted to place his party's stamp on the legislation by adding drug coverage. The point is that virtually nothing happens on Capitol Hill in a vacuum; every event must be placed in a context of a broader, more complex field of action.

Throughout the lengthy congressional process, many Republicans also supported an expansion of the government's involvement in health care. The final bill won approval in the House and Senate by votes of 328 to 72 and 86 to 11, respectively. Senator Robbert [sic] Packwood of Oregon, a senior Republican who chaired the Finance Committee when the GOP held the majority, described the emotionalism that colored the debate over a catastrophic-illness benefit at the first of three committee hearings in early 1987:

> I came to the Senate in 1969. I have been here through Carswell and Haynsworth [two unsuccessful Nixon nominees to the U.S. Supreme Court] and the invasion of Cambodia, President Nixon and Watergate, and President Carter's malaise, and now President Reagan and Iran and the Contras. I have seen issues rise and fall. . . . In those 17 years . . . I have not encountered an issue that engenders as much sympathy and feeling and heartache as the issue of catastrophic health costs, and it is uniform in Oregon or Texas or Missouri, Arkansas, or anyplace else.

Packwood's description conveyed the political appeal inherent in broadening health insurance coverage, but subsequent congressional action also showed a tough-mindedness in regard to the elderly that has been largely absent in the past. That attitude emerged when Congress endorsed Reagan's decision to require the elderly to pay for the benefit and then added an income-related supplemental premium to finance the expanded benefits. Congress also agreed implicitly with Reagan's decision not to consider at this stage the needs of people under 65 who may also lack coverage for catastrophic costs, although providing such coverage seemed to be part of the President's early directive to Bowen.

Federal policy makers regard the elderly as the most powerful private interest group in the health arena; as a consequence, they are particularly attentive to the pressures exerted by older people and their lobbies. A growing chorus of complaints by elderly citizens over the new tax is being heard in congressional offices. Thus, the resolve of Congress to require the elderly to pay for these benefits will be tested this year and beyond. At this point the AARP, which reluctantly accepted the new supplemental premium in the absence of a politically viable alternative, is striving to persuade its 30-million-member constituency that the new benefit represents a solid value for their money. Although there seems little likelihood that Congress will overhaul its approach to financing these new Medicare benefits, given the problems of the federal budget and the absence of politically viable financing alternatives, the controversy it is arousing will certainly influence the policy options under consideration when legislation on long-term care moves to center stage in 1989.

REFERENCES

1. Christensen S, Kasten R. Covering catastrophic expenses under Medicare. Health Aff (Millwood) 1988;7(5):79-93.

2. Rich S. Catastrophic insurance attacked as unfair tax. Washington Post. January 15, 1989:3.

Editor's Note

In the essay which follows, Fulda and Wilford comment forcefully on the legacy of the Task Force Report. Their essay should perhaps have been placed at the beginning rather than near the end of the collection. In either place, their comments are compelling.

Following the Fulda/Wilford essay is the previously unpublished final report of a project designed to provide a framework for evaluating the effects of managed care on the pharmaceutical marketplace–prospective road map at the end of this retrospective survey.

[Haworth co-indexing entry note]: "Editor's Note." Smith, Mickey C. Co-published simultaneously in *Journal of Research in Pharmaceutical Economics* (Pharmaceutical Products Press, an imprint of The Haworth Press, Inc.) Vol. 10, No. 4, 2001, p. 229; and: *Prescription Drugs Under Medicare: The Legacy of the Task Force on Prescription Drugs* (ed: Mickey C. Smith) Pharmaceutical Products Press, an imprint of The Haworth Press, Inc., 2001, p. 229. Single or multiple copies of this article are available for a fee from The Haworth Document Delivery Service [1-800-342-9678, 9:00 a.m. - 5:00 p.m. (EST). E-mail address: getinfo@haworthpressinc.com].

The Legacy of the HEW Task Force
on Prescription Drugs

Thomas R. Fulda
Bonnie B. Wilford

It has been nearly 35 years since the Medicare Program was enacted without including coverage for outpatient prescription drugs. In the intervening years, there have been a number of attempts, as President Lyndon Johnson did in January 1967, to focus the attention of the nation on the problems faced by elderly Americans in paying for the prescriptions they need. There have also been a number of failed legislative attempts, most notably the Medicare Catastrophic Coverage Act of 1988, to add outpatient drug coverage to Medicare. In January 1999, in his State of the Union Address to Congress, President Clinton again raised the issue of the ability of senior citizens to pay for their prescription drugs and proposed Medicare reforms which would include an outpatient prescription benefit. Whether the fate of this latest effort will be any different from that of its predecessors is yet to be determined.

There is reason to be pessimistic. The nation's capital is a place where all too often experience is ignored as the wheel is reinvented and studies are used to give the appearance of action when the resolve to solve a problem is absent. It is tempting to file the highly regarded reports of the HEW Task Force on Prescription Drugs, which com-

---

Thomas R. Fulda is Program Director, Drug Utilization Review, U.S. Pharmacopeia, 12601 Twinbrook Parkway, Rockville, MD 20852. Bonnie B. Wilford is Editor, *Pharmaceutical Policy Review.*

[Haworth co-indexing entry note]: "The Legacy of the HEW Task Force on Prescription Drugs." Fulda, Thomas R., and Bonnie B. Wilford. Co-published simultaneously in *Journal of Research in Pharmaceutical Economics* (Pharmaceutical Products Press, an imprint of The Haworth Press, Inc.) Vol. 10, No. 4, 2001, pp. 231-234; and: *Prescription Drugs Under Medicare: The Legacy of the Task Force on Prescription Drugs* (ed: Mickey C. Smith) Pharmaceutical Products Press, an imprint of The Haworth Press, Inc., 2001, pp. 231-234. Single or multiple copies of this article are available for a fee from The Haworth Document Delivery Service [1-800-342-9678, 9:00 a.m. - 5:00 p.m. (EST). E-mail address: getinfo@haworthpressinc.com].

pleted its work 30 years ago, among the legion studies that are gathering dust on bookshelves or have been discarded and forgotten.

Yet anyone willing and able to review the Task Force documents will discover among its findings statements that are as relevant to today's debate as they were when they were first released in 1969. The drafters of the Task Force offered the following timeless pearls:

- The requirements for appropriate prescription drug therapy by the elderly are very great–far greater, in fact, than those of any other group–and many elderly men and women are now unable to meet those needs with their limited incomes, savings, or present insurance coverage.
- Their inability to afford the drugs they require may well be reflected, in needless sickness and disability, unemployability, and hospitalization which could have been prevented by adequate out-of-hospital treatment.
- In order to improve the access of the elderly to high quality health care, and to protect them where possible against high drug expenses . . . there is a need for an out of hospital drug insurance program under Medicare.
- Rational prescribing, with due regard to quality of health care as well as to program costs, can be improved through cooperation of physicians, pharmacists, drug manufacturers, and a governmental agency.
- Reasonable program costs appear to be associated with (a) the use of a formulary developed by or in cooperation with the medical community, (b) the use of co-payment or co-insurance, (c) the use of utilization review procedures to prevent or minimize irrational prescribing, (d) the use of appropriate electronic or other data processing methods. . . . (e) simplified determination of beneficiary eligibility, (f) population coverage which obviates the adverse selection of high risk beneficiaries.
- In order to achieve the maximum benefits with whatever funds may be available, and to give maximum help to those of the elderly whose drug needs are the most burdensome, particular consideration should be given to providing coverage at the outset mainly for those prescription drugs which are most likely to be essential in the treatment of serious long term illness.

Clearly the particular issues faced and the environment explored by the HEW Task Force in the late 1960's was different from the cluster of issues and the environment in which a Medicare outpatient prescription drug benefit is being considered in the late 1990's. The intervening years have seen globalization and significant consolidation of the pharmaceutical industry and the emergence of managed care as a major force in health care. Drugs have become more expensive and much more important in the treatment of disease. Thanks to the Internet, consumers have access to more information about prescription drugs and other health care information than ever before. And–more to the point of this discussion–outpatient prescription insurance is more readily available than it was 30 years ago but still beyond the reach of many seniors.

Reflecting on these changes, the Office of the Assistant Secretary for Planning and Evaluation at the Department of Health and Human Services awarded a contract in 1996 to the Pharmaceutical Policy Project at the George Washington University Center for Health Policy Research to reexamine the questions first raised by the HEW Task Force and to develop a framework for research and evaluation into the effects of managed care on the pharmaceutical marketplace.

Working in consultation with an advisory panel that was broadly representative of the health care delivery system, project staff examined much of the relevant scholarly literature of the past 30 years, as well as other sources of information that would shed light on how the health care system could have evolved so far without finding a way to cover a component so important as prescription drugs. In pursuing their deliberations, staff and advisors were guided by two global questions: (1) What do we know about the pharmaceutical marketplace and the ways it has evolved in response to managed care? and (2) What do we not know that we need to know? Over the two-year span of the project, "what we know" was documented in literature reviews and a database. Perhaps more usefully, "what we do not know" was framed in a series of questions, such as:

- What is the difference, if any, between *access* to prescription drug benefits and benefits actually *used*? What is the significance of such a difference?
- When pharmacy benefits are purchased by employers or the government, do the needs of the purchasers take precedence over those of the patients? Is managed care different from fee-for-ser-

vice arrangements in this regard? To what extent do decisions by purchasers influence providers and care provided to consumers?

- How does a plan's ability to meet consumer *expectations*, as opposed to consumer needs, affect patient satisfaction? How do patients assess the quality of their care versus the quality of their lives?

Finally, in reading the materials from the HEW Task Force on Prescription Drugs, the "Framework for Research and Evaluation into the Effects of Managed Care on the Pharmaceutical Marketplace," and the other documents in this collection, we hope that you will emerge more enlightened than when you started. Where this is a more rational and ordered world we would hope that the issues raised in these documents would be appropriately addressed during the current debate about a Medicare drug benefit. Realism and experience suggest to us that this is unlikely to happen. History may repeat itself and fear of the costs of providing a drug benefit and the clash of the interests involved in the political process may again leave us with the problem unsolved. Perhaps the most that can be expected is a Medicare drug benefit, however imperfect, that will set off another cycle of effort to answer the questions that have been and should be asked by researchers and policy makers alike. We fervently hope so.

A Framework
for Research and Evaluation
into the Effects of Managed Care
on the Pharmaceutical Marketplace:
Excerpts from the Final Report

Advisory Panel on DHHS DO16*

*Members of the Advisory Panel: James R. Allen, M.D., M.P.H.; Calvin J. Anthony, Pharm.D.; Lynn A. Bosco, M.D., M.P.H.; Laurie Beth Burke, R.Ph., M.P.H.; Patricia J. Byrns, M.D.; Cheryl Austein Casnoff (Senior Government Project Officer); David Clark, R.Ph., M.B.A.; Burke Fishburn, M.P.P. (Government Project Officer); Thomas R. Fulda; Jean-Paul Gagnon, R.Ph., Ph.D.; Linda F. Golodner; Kathleen Gondek, Ph.D.; Henry Grabowski, Ph.D.; Charles R. Grezlak, Ph.D.; David J. Gross, Ph.D.; Eric Katz, J.D.; Arthur Lawrence, M.D., M.P.H.; Helene L. Lipton, Ph.D.; Lucinda L. Maine, Ph.D.; Julie Matsumoto, M.S.T.H.; Patrick L. McKercher, R.Ph., Ph.D.; Michael Miller, M.D.; Louis Morris, Ph.D.; Mark Novitch, M.D. (Principal Investigator); Francis B. Palumbo, Ph.D., J.D.; Peter M. Penna, Pharm.D.; Gary S. Persinger; Michael Pollard, J.D., M.P.H.; T. Donald Rucker, Ph.D.; Claudia Schur, Ph.D.; Stuart O. Schweitzer, Ph.D.; David G. Schulke; Kevin A. Schulman, M.D.; Robert C. Seidman, M.P.H.; Sheila A. Shulman, L.L.B., M.P.H.; Betsy L. Sleath, Ph.D., R.Ph.; Janice Whitehouse; Bonnie B. Wilford (Project Director); Karen Williams; and Raymond L. Woosley, M.D., Ph.D. Opinions and recommendations offered by members of the Advisory Panel are their own and do not necessarily represent those of the organizations with which they are (or were) affiliated.

Acknowledgment: Prepared by the Pharmaceutical Policy Project at The George Washington University under DHHS DO16, contract number 282-92-0040 with the Office of the Assistant Secretary for Planning and Evaluation, Department of Health and Human Services; Burke Fishburn, M.P.P., Project Officer; Mark Novitch, M.D., Principal Investigator.

[Haworth co-indexing entry note]: "A Framework for Research and Evaluation into the Effects of Managed Care on the Pharmaceutical Marketplace: Excerpts from the Final Report." Advisory Panel on DHHS DO16. Co-published simultaneously in *Journal of Research in Pharmaceutical Economics* (Pharmaceutical Products Press, an imprint of The Haworth Press, Inc.) Vol. 10, No. 4, 2001, pp. 235-266; and: *Prescription Drugs Under Medicare: The Legacy of the Task Force on Prescription Drugs* (ed: Mickey C. Smith) Pharmaceutical Products Press, an imprint of The Haworth Press, Inc., 2001, pp. 235-266. Single or multiple copies of this article are available for a fee from The Haworth Document Delivery Service [1-800-342-9678, 9:00 a.m. - 5:00 p.m. (EST). E-mail address: getinfo@haworthpressinc.com].

FINAL REPORT

Since the discovery of aspirin at the turn of the century, advances in both scientific understanding and technology have enabled pharmaceutical researchers to target successively more complex diseases. Focus on tissue biochemistry provided insights that led to the successful development of antibiotics. As antibiotics enabled people to survive to more advanced ages, researchers focused on cell biochemistry to find cures for more complex, chronic diseases. . . .

Pharmaceutical discoveries since the 1950s have revolutionized therapy for chronic as well as acute conditions. . . . Had no progress been made against disease between 1960 and 1990, roughly 335,000 more people would have died in 1990 alone (PhRMA, 1997).

Numerous studies have shown that use of pharmaceuticals within a continuum of care is highly cost-effective (Figure 1). Yet little is known about how the emergence of managed care has affected the development and marketing of pharmaceutical products and consumers' access to pharmaceutical therapies and related services. . . .

Competing demands to control health care costs, improve access to services and provide a high quality of care are creating powerful and often conflicting pressures on the nation's health care system (Knickman, Hughes, Taylor et al., 1996). It is clear that the system is experiencing profound change. While most observers agree that managed care is central to this transformation, it is not the only producer of change. Researchers point out that events as disparate as welfare reform and the federal Balanced Budget Amendment on the one hand, and advances in medical technology, gene mapping and understanding of neuroscience on the other, all affect the organization and delivery of health care services. Among the most dramatic of these changes is the remarkable growth of managed care and the burgeoning competition among large health care systems (Rosenbaum & Richards, 1996; Curtiss, 1986).

Sorting out these influences and developing a better understanding of the effects of managed care on the pharmaceutical marketplace are essential to achieving an accurate understanding of the current situation and developing a clear projection of the types of policy research that will be needed to manage such change in a positive way.

FIGURE 1. Drop in Death Rate for Diseases Treated with Pharmaceuticals, 1965-1995.

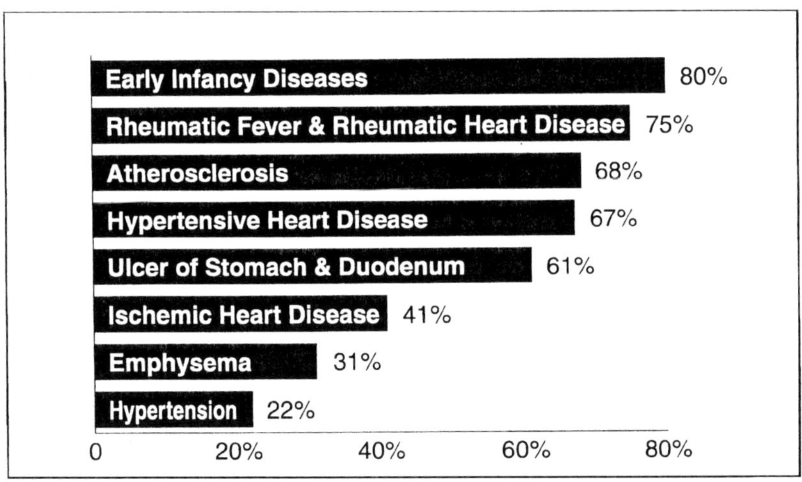

Source: Pharmaceutical Research and Manufacturers of America (PhRMA) (1997). 1997 Industry Profile. Washington, DC: PhRMA, p. 7. Reprinted by permission.

The implications of such an understanding are significant for all the stakeholders. For pharmaceutical producers, managed care organizations, and purchasers of care, huge amounts of money are at stake. For health professionals of all disciplines–but particularly for physicians and pharmacists–practice changes will either enhance or diminish their ability to deliver high-quality care. For patients, health and life are in the balance. . . .

THE PHARMACEUTICAL INDUSTRY

As with other sectors of the economy, the U.S. pharmaceutical industry is undergoing profound changes that influence how it develops and markets products (Boston Consulting Group, 1993). These changes have come about in response to a number of factors, including the globalization of the pharmaceutical industry and its markets, the consolidation of the U.S. health care industry, the explosive growth of managed care arrangements, greater sophistication on the part of purchasers, and the aging of consumer populations in all developed countries (PhRMA, 1997).

Research and Development: The pharmaceutical industry is, as Pollard (1990) characterizes it, "rooted in the soil of innovation; new products, preferably patentable, are its cash crop." Within the past decade, pharmaceutical products have become a much more potent element in modern medical intervention, but have achieved visibility with policymakers primarily because of attendant high costs. Manufacturers counter criticisms by advancing the argument that the development of new drugs is a costly and risky enterprise, pointing out that only five of about 5,000 substances screened in preclinical studies actually progress to human testing. Of these five, only one makes it to the pharmacy shelves. Thus, the prices of "successful" drugs must compensate also for the costs of the research and development of the "unsuccessful" drugs, i.e., those that do not make it to the marketplace (Moore, 1996).

With U.S. manufacturers investing an amount equivalent to 19 percent of sales back into new product R&D (PhRMA website, 1997), the pharmaceutical industry is among a small number of U.S. industries that invest heavily in the future (Grabowski & Vernon, 1990, 1994; BCG, 1996). These investments reflect both the time and intensity of effort required for approval of new drug applications (NDAs) submitted to the Food and Drug Administration (BCG, 1996).

BCG investigators developed the concept of the "cycle of innovation" to explain the increasing cost of breakthrough drugs, by relating the products to points on a continuum of desired results (Figure 2). These range from palliation of symptoms, to control of disease mechanisms, and finally to cure or prevention. Examining the industry's current position in the cycle with respect to a number of major medical illnesses (such as diabetes, many forms of cancer, and HIV disease, for example) the BCG analysts posit that some of the most common diseases treatable with pharmacotherapies are at the highest-cost (cure or prevention) stage in the cycle of innovation (BCG, 1993).

Approval Processes: A more flexible regulatory approach for breakthrough drugs has evolved over the past decade (DiMasi, 1996). This is reflected in regulations for early access programs and for accelerated approval based on changes in surrogate endpoints (Shulman & Brown, 1995). Indeed, median drug approval times

FIGURE 2. The Cycle of Innovation.

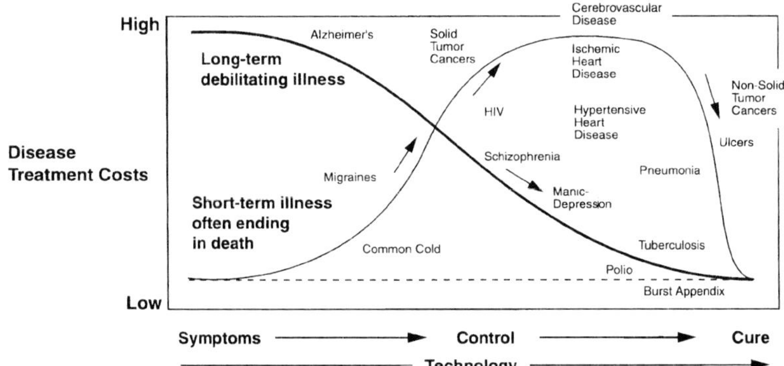

Source: Boston Consulting Group (1993). The Contribution of Pharmaceutical Companies: What's at Stake for America. Boston, MA: The Boston Consulting Group, Inc., p. 10. Reprinted by permission.

declined by more than half over the decade ending in 1996 (Friedman, 1997a). Recent figures are even more dramatic. For drug and biologic applications first submitted in 1996, approval times currently average 12 months, which is a third less time than was required for 1993 submissions (Friedman, 1997b). FDA reform legislation enacted in late 1997 aimed at sustaining these trends while maintaining the agency's historic focus on patient protection.

Horizontal Integration: Pharmaceutical manufacturers have reacted to these changes by allocating more resources to research, particularly for geriatric products, and by expanding marketing activities geared toward managed care clients. Discounted prices, especially to large customers such as hospital systems and HMOs, are occurring throughout the health care industry. Also, a number of major mergers have been completed over the past several years, thereby enhancing the capacity of the "new" companies to compete across several product lines both domestically and globally. It has been suggested that such mergers of pharmaceutical manufacturers produce economies of scale that optimize the time and resources required for innovation (DiMasi, Grabowski & Vernon, 1995). Additional integration likely will arise from manufacturers' ventures into disease management programs (Etheredge, 1995; KPMG Peat Marwick, 1996), which are population-based approaches that integrate multiple tasks of risk identification, intervention, and assessment of outcomes (Epstein & McGlynn, 1997).

DiMasi, Grabowski and Vernon (1995) examined the relationships among firm size, R&D costs, and output in the pharmaceutical industry. In a survey of 12 U.S.-owned pharmaceutical companies, they found that the R&D cost per new drug approved decreased as firm size increased, while sales per new drug increased in parallel with firm size. Because of the economies of scale in pharmaceutical R&D, as well as the fixed nature of the industry's R&D costs, the authors concluded that, in principle, larger firms can spread these fixed costs over more projects and also over a larger expected sales base. In a review of the effects of industry consolidation on research and development and product innovation, Gagnon (1996) predicted that future pharmaceutical "research and development will focus on unmet medical needs, breakthrough drugs, drug delivery systems, and drugs not susceptible to therapeutic substitution."

Vertical Integration: Various forms of vertical integration between pharmaceutical manufacturers and pharmacy benefit managers (PBMs) have been achieved (Shulman, Healy & Lasagna, 1997). These alignments take a variety of forms, ranging from acquisitions to contractual agreements that cover collaboration on patient and physician education programs, joint development of patient compliance strategies, or the formation of new companies to develop disease management protocols (Armstrong, 1996; Nagy, 1995).

A close relationship with a managed care organization can help a drugmaker carve a niche in the developing field of disease management because of the need to focus on patient populations rather than individual patients. Such programs require "the development of clear clinical guidelines, agreement on the part of providers and patients to participate, a sophisticated information architecture, well-designed and tested interventions and a logical measurement plan for the collection of outcomes" data (Epstein & McGlynn, 1997)–all tasks within the purview of managed care.

Pricing Policies: As managed care plans use their substantial buying power to alter purchasing patterns in the marketplace, an area of potential backlash against these arrangements is evident in a series of legislative and court battles over unitary pricing (referred to as "anti-discriminatory pricing" bills by supporters and "anti-discount pricing" by opponents). These proposals typically require that pharmaceutical manufacturers and distributors offer their products to all retail purchasers on the same terms and conditions. They generally allow only price differentials that reflect: (1) reductions justified by economies or efficiencies realized through volume purchases; (2) reductions available through market share agreements; (3) reductions for placing a drug on a formulary; (4) reductions for prompt payment; (5) reductions for limited site delivery; or (6) opportunities involving free merchandise, samples, or similar trade concessions. Thus, the concept is favored by independent and chain pharmacies that generally are excluded from the most favorable discount schemes, and opposed by mail service and managed care pharmacies that are their principal beneficiaries. . . .

Drug Costs: Members of the Advisory Panel predicted that prescription drug costs will continue to rise, albeit at a slowed rate, regardless of the cost containment tools employed by managed care plans, for two reasons. First, neither modern medicine nor managed care has reduced the percentage of ill people in the population. In fact, advances in clinical care actually increases this percentage by keeping more people alive, albeit not cured. The protease inhibitors and other drugs for the treatment of HIV disease are a striking example of this point.

Second, society has expanded the concept of health to encompass palliation of an array of psychological and physical problems (infertility, panic attacks) that in the past were seen either as not medical problems or as not treatable. Pharmacotherapies now exist for many of these conditions, and the demand to use them probably will overwhelm most efforts to restrict access.

Responses to Managed Care: While not yet supported with published studies, widespread anecdotal reports suggest that drugmakers are deciding against pursuing promising research because of their belief that managed care practices render the market potential insufficient to support certain drugs under prevailing economic conditions (Grabowski, 1994). The extent to which such a belief is accurate is not yet clear. However, in a study for the National Bureau of Economics, Cutler and Sheiner (1997) found preliminary evidence that managed care has reduced the rate of diffusion of new medical technologies.

Genuardi, Stiller and Trapnell (1996) maintain that two characteristics render the pharmaceutical industry particularly vulnerable to pressure from managed care: (1) the proliferation of generic and brand-name drugs that can be substituted for other drugs in the same class; and (2) the fixed-cost structure of the pharmaceutical industry, in which the front-end investment in R&D and smaller marginal production costs make it worthwhile for manufacturers to pay rebates to those organizations capable of shifting market share . . . (Figure 3).

Summers and Gumbhir (1991) queried a group of pharmaceutical industry executives and pharmacy educators about the future effects of managed care on the research-intensive pharmaceutical industry. The respondents said that they anticipated new approaches to drug product development and marketing, as well as cost-effectiveness and quality of life studies. The drug company executives in particular predicted a much stronger emphasis on costs under managed care, and therefore foresaw the need for research that can demonstrate the economic value of new pharmaceuticals. . . .

MANAGED CARE

While the term "managed care" lacks a commonly accepted definition and has been used to characterize a wide variety of health care plans, Dacso and Dacso (1996) have characterized its essential attributes as involving: (1) contractual arrangements with selected providers, such as pharmacies and pharmacists, who furnish a package of services to enrollees for a predetermined fee (capitation); (2) imposition of criteria for selection of providers, such as board certification or accreditation; (3) application of quality assurance, utilization review, and outcome measures; (4) use of financial or program coverage incentives or penalties to direct enrollees toward certain providers and away from others; (5) provider participation in risk-sharing; and (6) management of providers to assure that enrollees or members receive "appropriate" care from a cost-efficient mix of providers. . . .

Pharmacy Benefit Managers (PBMs): Pharmacy benefit managers were active even before the concept of managed care took hold for prescription drug benefits (Genuardi, Stiller & Trapnell, 1996). The influence of these specialized benefits administrators has grown steadily in the 1990s (OIG, 1997; DeNoon, 1996), with PBMs currently managing prescription drug benefits for more than 35 million enrollees (Novartis, 1997b) (see Figure 4).

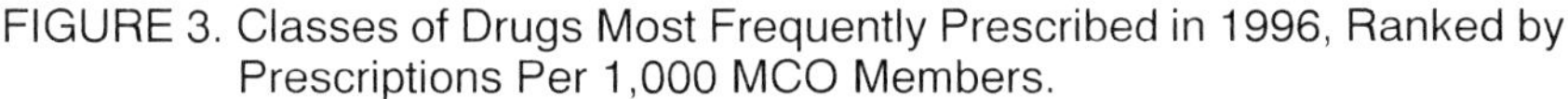

FIGURE 3. Classes of Drugs Most Frequently Prescribed in 1996, Ranked by Prescriptions Per 1,000 MCO Members.

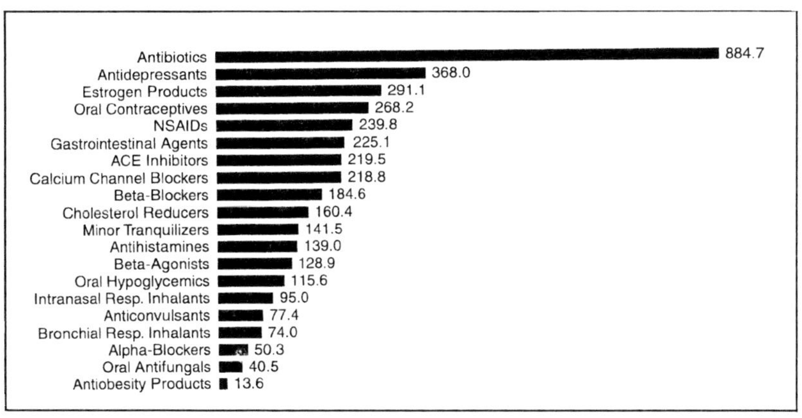

Source: Novartis (1997). The Novartis Pharmacy Benefit Report: Facts & Figures, 1997 Edition. East Hanover, NJ: Novartis Pharmaceuticals Corporation, p. 27. Reprinted by permission.

Although several dozen PBMs are active in the marketplace, a handful of firms dominate. Data from the Health Care Financing Administration (HCFA, 1997) suggest that, in 1995, the five largest PBMs managed benefits for 80 percent of all health plan enrollees served by PBMs. In fact, three-fourths of the 263 MCOs that responded to a recent survey by the DHHS Office of the Inspector General reported that they contract with PBMs; this number has nearly tripled since 1993 (OIG, 1997). A larger proportion (77 percent) of the unaffiliated, local MCOs reported using PBMs than did the local affiliates of national or regional MCOs (46 percent). The OIG survey further found that a majority of the MCOs that use PBMs serve Medicare and/or Medicaid beneficiaries (74 percent); contract with one of the five largest PBMs, each of which is owned by or allied with drug manufacturers (52 percent); and are for-profit plans (61 percent).

Gagnon (1996) cites two principal reasons for the rapid growth of PBMs: (1) the widespread acceleration of cost-containment efforts due to public anxiety over escalating health care costs and (2) the equally widespread adoption of computers to manage all sorts of data, including health care data, which permit the standardization of treatment protocols and prices. Shulman, Healy and Lasagna (1997)

FIGURE 4. Use of PBM Services, by Type of Service.

A 1997 report by the DHHS Office of the Inspector General described Pharmacy Benefit Management services as falling into three categories. The percentage of managed care plans and other purchasers using each type of service is shown in parentheses.

1.   *Basic services*, which are composed of system management functions. These include:

    (94%)   *Claims processing*, involving processing individual prescription claims for payment. This may involve confirming the patient's eligibility and the conformance of the drug with the plan's formulary.

    (74%)   *On-line pharmacy networks*, which employ an electronic link between independent pharmacies and the PBM for the transmission of claims, as well as to adjudicate eligibility and payment decisions on behalf of a given health plan.

    (46%)   *Mail service pharmacies*, which involve dispensing of prescriptions for chronic conditions by mail service pharmacies rather than through traditional retail pharmacy settings.

2.   *Intermediate services*, which harness the economic leverage of the PBM and its capacity to screen large databases of prescription claims against utilization and quality criteria. Such services include:

    (84%)   *Drug use review services* involve scrutiny of individual prescriptions and overall prescribing patterns in comparison with pre-determined cost and/or quality criteria. *Prospective review* screens individual prescriptions before they are filled to identify quality or utilization problems. *Retrospective review*, which occurs after prescriptions are filled and the claims submitted for payment, involves screening large numbers of claims to identify patterns of inappropriate prescribing or dispensing, potentially fraudulent activity, or patient compliance problems.

    (71%)   *Formulary development and management services* involve using the PBM to evaluate and select the drugs to be included on the health plan's lists of preferred drugs (formularies). In such cases, the PBM decides which drugs to include in the formulary, as well as the relative preference ranking for each drug. In some cases, PBMs also actively manage prescription drug formularies on behalf of health plans. In this role, they typically handle requests for prior authorization; manage limits on the frequency or number of prescriptions or refills allowed; and enforce guidelines for generic or therapeutic substitution programs.

    (56%)   *Educational interventions* involve contact with physicians, pharmacists, and patients to alter product selection, consumption and related practices.

3.   *Enhanced services*, which are the most recently developed, involve PBMs in directly managing patient care. They include:

    (35%)   *Disease management practices*, which are designed to manage the treatment of groups of patients who are grouped by diagnosis. Disease management is particularly popular in the management of chronic conditions, in which drug therapy is expected to be needed on a long-term basis.

    (28%)   *Outcomes/cost-effectiveness research* using the PBM's database for research on the cost-effectiveness or outcomes of drug selections and therapies.

Source: Office of the Inspector General (1997). Experiences of Health Maintenance Organizations with Pharmacy Benefit Management Companies (OEI-01-95-00110). Washington, DC: OIG, April, p. 7.

point out that it is this ability of PBMs to switch or limit prescriptions–thereby constraining physician prescribing behavior and consumer choice–that is the key to their competitive edge.

Concerns about the effect of PBMs on the operations of pharmacy programs led HCFA to commission a major study (Kreling, Lipton, Collins & Hertz, 1996). Concerns have intensified because of the ownership and/or contractual relationships that exist between some PBMs and pharmaceutical manufacturers, and the absence of research-based evaluations of the effects of such arrangements (Schulman, Rubenstein, Abernethy et al., 1996). Questions of conflict of interest have been raised, as have issues related to potential anti-competitive trade practices associated with the mergers; the latter have been examined by the Federal Trade Commission (OIG, 1997). On the other hand, Shulman and Brown (1996) have reported that the presence of PBMs in the marketplace has increased the level of price competition among pharmaceutical manufacturers and distributors, although the effects of this change are not well understood. Moreover, PBMs' use of integrative "disease management" concepts, research-based clinical protocols and patient education services have been widely remarked as holding the promise of improved care and patient outcomes (KPMG Peat Marwick, 1996; Nash, 1995). . . .

Sources and Methods of Payment for Prescription Drugs Under Managed Care

Spending on outpatient prescription drugs was nearly $73 billion for 2.2 billion prescriptions in 1996, up from $21 billion in 1985. The proportion of these costs borne by third-party payers was 58 percent, as compared with 45 percent in 1985 (Novartis, 1997a) (Figure 5).

The 1997 OIG report noted that "Medicare and Medicaid beneficiaries together constitute the largest segments of the outpatient prescription drug market." Although prescription drugs are an optional benefit, every state Medicaid program incorporates outpatient prescription drug coverage. The Medicare program, on the other had, has limited its outpatient drug coverage to a few categories of drugs, such as immunosuppressants and cancer drugs. However, a significant number of indigent patients have dual eligibility for the Medicare and Medicaid programs. Moreover, Medicare is indirectly supporting broader outpatient prescription drug coverage, as its risk-based MCOs rely on this benefit to attract Medicare enrollees (OIG, 1997).

Sources of Payment: Sources of payment for prescription drugs purchased in retail outlets have changed dramatically since 1980, when 66 percent of drugs were paid for out-of-pocket, 32 percent via private health insurance and Medicaid; in 1996, these numbers were 41 percent and 59 percent, respectively (Novartis, 1997a; Genuardi, Stiller & Trapnell, 1996). Even with this level of third-party payment, however, consumers are less sheltered from the burden of paying for drugs than for other services (Comanor & Schweitzer, 1995).

Methods of Payment: Capitation, which has been defined as a fixed payment for a defined set of services (Christensen & Fassett, 1996), is one of the defining characteristics and most controversial aspects of managed care. In fee-for-service health plans, the bulk of the financial risk for the cost of services delivered falls on the insurer (or employer, in self-insured plans). Under capitation, on the other hand, part of the financial risk is shifted to the provider, who has agreed to provide a predetermined panel of services for a fixed cost. The degree to which risk is shared depends on the particular method of capitation used. Under fully capitated arrangements, all services are delivered under a single comprehensive package (Nash, 1995). Such shifting of risk provides an incentive for the provider to be more cost-conscious, which ideally leads to greater emphasis on preventive services and attention to outcomes. On the other hand, it also can lead to underuse of essential services or to substitution of one therapy for a more preferred intervention largely on the basis of cost.

FIGURE 5. Sources of Payment for Prescription Drugs.

	Dollars			Prescriptions		
	Dollars (000s)	**% of Class**	**% of Total US Retail**	**Rxs (000s)**	**% of Class**	**% of Total US Retail**
Total All Payment Types	2,893,713	100.0%	6.8%	69,136	100.0%	6.5%
Third-Party	1,657,199	57.3%	6.3%	40,119	58.0%	6.5%
Medicaid Non-Third-Party	290,462	10.0%	6.0%	6,310	9.1%	5.7%
Cash	946,051	32.7%	8.1%	22,707	32.8%	6.8%

Managed Care Cost Containment

Gross (1995) has classified the methods used by MCOs in their pursuit of cost containment as manufacturer-based approaches, market-based approaches, physician- and pharmacy-based approaches, and patient-based approaches.

Manufacturer-based approaches include price regulations, discounting requirements and rebate programs. Such approaches have been applied by the Medicaid system since 1990 (Gross, 1995). There is considerable debate as to whether these approaches have a negative effect on manufacturer-based research and development and attendant product innovation (Berndt, 1994; Comanor and Schweitzer, 1995).

Market-based approaches involve the promotion of generic and therapeutic substitution and cost-effectiveness studies (Figure 6). They are in wide use in both the public and private sectors (Gross, 1995). Some commentators (Horn, Sharkey, Tracy et al., 1996) have asserted that limitations on the scope of available medications in managed care settings may result increased patient care costs for office consultations and hospitalizations that offset any savings achieved. However, the available data are inconclusive.

Physician- and pharmacy-based approaches include formularies, drug utilization review (DUR)–required by the Medicaid program since 1991–drug budgets, and limits on dispensing fees. These initiatives are intended to control prescription drug expenses, either by increasing physicians' and pharmacists' sensitivity to drug costs or by intervening directly in their decisionmaking processes (Soumerai & Lipton, 1995; Gross, 1995). Again, many of these cost-containment approaches predate or stem from the early development of managed care (Rucker, 1983; Curtiss, 1986).

Patient-based approaches frequently involve the use of cost-sharing (through deductibles, co-insurance, and copayments), which is designed to increase consumers' sensitivity to prescription drug prices (Gross, 1995). Most managed care plans also limit coverage to specific drugs or classes of drugs and the amount of drugs dispensed at one time. They also may impose limits on the number of refills per prescription, as well as the duration of time that a prescription is valid (Vogenberg, 1997a).

The long-term consequences of various cost-containment strategies are not well understood. Of the studies that assess short-term effects, the most significant finding is an observation of decreased drug

FIGURE 6. Utilization of Cost Containment Approaches, by MCO Model Type.

Cost-Containment Strategies	Staff	Group	IPA	Network	Overall
Generic Substitution	100.0%	90.0%	96.3%	90.9%	95.0%
DUE/DUR	100.0%	80.0%	92.6%	100.0%	93.3%
Guidelines	58.3%	60.0%	59.3%	72.7%	61.7%
Ther. Substitution	50.0%	80.0%	51.9%	45.5%	55.0%
Ther. Interchange	41.7%	80.0%	40.7%	36.4%	46.7%

Source: Novartis (1997). The Novartis Pharmacy Benefit Report: Facts & Figures, 1997 Edition, East Hanover, NJ: Novartis Pharmaceuticals Corporation, p. 13. Reprinted by permission.

utilization even at low levels of copayments. For example, studies by Reeder and Nelson (1985) and by Soumerai, Avorn and Ross-Degnan (1987) reported reductions in the use of both essential and nonessential drugs when a Medicaid copayment was introduced.

Some investigators (Buchanan, Leibowitz & Keesey, 1996; Horn, Sharkey and Tracy et al., 1996) have cautioned that a number of cost-containment approaches, particularly restrictive formularies, may raise rather than lower long-term patient care costs. (It should be noted, however, that the Horn study attracted criticism of the study methodology and the authors' conclusions.)

Other studies point to significant potential savings associated with use of cost containment strategies. For example, Knowlton and Knapp (1994) studied a group of community pharmacists over a nine-month period to assess the effects of pharmacist interventions to (1) enhance communication with patients and physicians, (2) to intervene in real or potential drug-related problems, and (3) to change prescribed medications to contain costs. The authors concluded that the pharmacist interventions enhanced patient satisfaction and reduced monthly prescription drug expenditures.

Similarly, little is known about the effects of managed care cost-containment approaches on the quality of health care (Bloom & Fendrick, 1996). Negative effects have been reported by Horn et al. (1996) and by Soumerai and colleagues. Soumerai and Lipton (1995) expressed concern that an unintended consequence of computer-based DUR based on inadequate evidence-based studies may lead to undertreatment. . . .

Soumerai, Ross-Degnan, Fortess et al. (1993) have argued that great improvements in research methodology are needed before definitive recommendations are possible about how to implement cost-control policies without compromising quality. Lasagna (1994) has pointed to the need for reliable data to address access issues, including the difficult problem of defining inappropriate versus appropriate medication use, and second-order effects on utilization of physician, other outpatient, and hospital services.

Populations Enrolled in Managed Care

The issue of whether and how consumers have access to care, as well as whether technical access translates into actual use of pharmacotherapies and related services, is a core question.

Slightly more than 52 percent of all Americans have some part of their health benefits administered through managed care arrangements (Novartis, 1997b), and it is likely that the percentage of Americans enrolled in managed care plans will continue to grow (Jensen, Morrisey, Gaffney et al., 1997) (Figure 7).

Enrollment and Disenrollment: While high levels of enrollee turnover marked the early days of managed care, recent data indicate

FIGURE 7. Enrollment in Managed Care, by MCO Model Type.

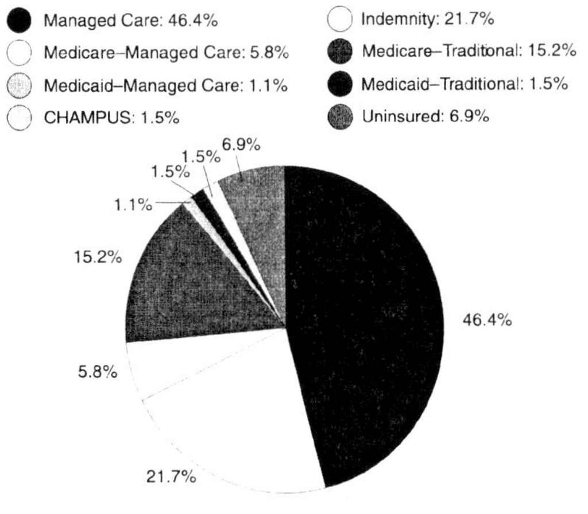

Percentages may not total 100% due to rounding.

Source: Norvartis (1997). The Novartis Pharmacy Benefit Report: Trends & Forecasts, 1997 Edition. East Hanover, NJ: Novartis Pharmaceuticals Corporation, p. 9. Reprinted by permission.

that time-in-plan is increasing (Novartis, 1997b). The average length of retention per member is projected to increase from 3.4 years in 1995 to 3.9 years in 1998 for persons with individual coverage; from 5.6 years in 1995 to 6.0 years in 1998 for persons enrolled in commercial/group health plans; and from 3.4 years in 1995 to 4.3 years in 1998 for Medicare enrollees (Novartis, 1997b).

A 1997 study by Families USA found that some managed care plans retain patients at a rate far higher than others. The Families USA study found annual rates of disenrollment that ranged from 2.4 percent for a managed care plan in Massachusetts to 81.1 percent for a plan in Florida. The study further found that nine of the 10 plans with the highest retention rates were not-for-profit, while seven of the 10 plans with the lowest retention rates were for-profit. (Plan retention rates have important implications for research, because adjusting for periods of disenrollment is difficult and complicates many analyses of treatment patterns, costs, and interventions.)

Geographic Distribution: Managed care enrollment varies across geographic regions as certain states and large employers actively encourage or discourage growth through legislative and administrative initiatives (Rodwin, 1996). A 1996 survey for *Business Insurance* magazine led to the prediction that approximately 50 percent of the population of the Southwestern and Mid-Atlantic states will be enrolled in managed care by the year 2000, while only 25 percent of residents of the South Central states will be. . . .

Sociodemographic Factors: Overall, MCOs tend to enroll a younger but not much healthier population than traditional fee-for-service plans. For example, a study using 1989 data from the National Medical Expenditure Survey found that managed care enrollees tend to be families with children under the age of 19, whereas enrollees in fee-for-service plans were less likely to be families with children. The authors speculate that younger families may be more willing to join managed care plans because they have not yet formed strong ties to their physicians (Taylor, Beauregard & Vistnes, 1995). Conversely, older patients may be unwilling to sever long-standing relationships established with physicians under fee-for-service plans (Hellinger, 1995).

Poverty status is an important independent predictor of managed care enrollment. Taylor and colleagues found that in 1989, "near poor" individuals were less likely than those with higher incomes to enroll in a managed care plan (Taylor, Beauregard & Vistnes, 1995).

Some studies suggest that race may interact with age as a special variable (Taylor, Beauregard & Vistnes, 1995; Ware, Bayliss, Rogers, et al., 1996). In a study conducted to examine determinants of the use of medications by elderly African-American and white community residents, Fillenbaum, Hanlon, Corder et al. (1993) found that although the health status of the African-Americans appeared to be similar to that of the whites, the African-American study subjects used fewer drugs, either prescription or nonprescription. Using NMES data to study the care of children, Hahn (1995) examined the relationship between minority status and the use of prescription medicines. He found that African-American and Hispanic children tended to receive fewer prescriptions than whites and were less likely to actually obtain and use the medicines prescribed. . . .

Prescription Drug Benefits: Ninety-five percent of persons enrolled in a managed care plan in 1996 had some sort of prescription drug benefit (Novartis, 1997a) (Figure 8). MCOs surveyed by Novartis reported spending an average $14.26 per member per month for prescription drugs in 1996; this represented an increase of $2.63 over 1995.

Effects on Consumer Access To and Use of Prescription Drugs

Given the popularity of various administrative restrictions on prescription drug benefits in publicly funded and some private health

FIGURE 8. Distribution of Populations with Prescription Drug Coverage.

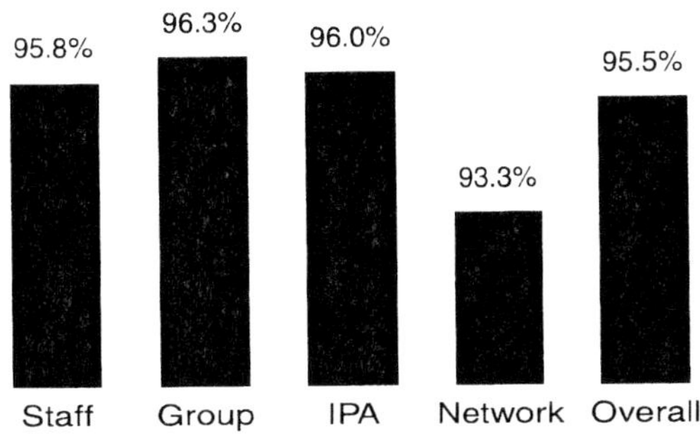

Source: Novartis (1997). The Novartis Pharmacy Benefit Report: Facts & Figures, 1997 Edition. East Hanover, NJ: Novartis Pharmaceuticals Corporation, p. 7. Reprinted by permission.

plans (which predates the advent of managed care), it is remarkable how little information is available to answer important questions about the effects of such restrictions on utilization, expenditures, and health outcomes (Weiner, Lyles, Steinwachs et al., 1991). The literature that exists is divided in its conclusions.

Drug Utilization Review: Critics of DUR suggest that its benefits have not been substantiated (Soumerai & Lipton, 1995). Other authors conclude that DUR programs are productive and that physician sensitivity to drug prices curbs inappropriately expensive prescribing (Hux & Naylor, 1994). To encourage research in this area, HCFA commissioned a study that has developed guidelines for evaluating the effects of DUR in the Medicaid program (Zimmerman, Collins, Lipowski et al., 1994).

Formularies: The literature on the effects of drug formularies also is inconclusive (Schweitzer & Shiota, 1992). One reason is that formularies differ markedly in degree of restrictiveness. Schweitzer, Salehi and Boling (1985) evaluated the impact of such restrictiveness by investigating the percent of newly approved drugs included in state Medicaid program formularies, and the time elapsed between FDA approval of those drugs and their appearance on the formularies. They found that the proportion of newly approved drugs appearing on state formularies ranged from 19 to 73 percent. The time lag from approval of the drugs to their inclusion in the formularies ranged from one to five years.

Using a slightly different approach, Grabowski (1988) found that, in six states studied, new drug products generally were available to Medicaid recipients during only two of the first five years following their approval by the FDA. Beyond duplicative products, the restricted drugs included products rated highly for medical importance by the FDA.

Effects of Cost Containment: The RAND Health Insurance Experiment (1985) directly examined the effects of benefit coverage on the consumption of prescription drugs. Study authors Leibowitz, Manning and Newhouse concluded that "individuals with more generous insurance buy more prescription drugs." On the other hand, a study of elderly persons found that modest increases in copayment amounts were not associated with a consistent change in use of prescription drugs for self-limiting and chronic conditions.

An equally important issue is that technical access to prescription drugs does not appear to be directly related to the number of medications actually used (Horn, Sharkey, Tracy et al., 1996) (Figure 9).

FIGURE 9. Prescriptions Per 1,000 MCO Members, by Model Type.

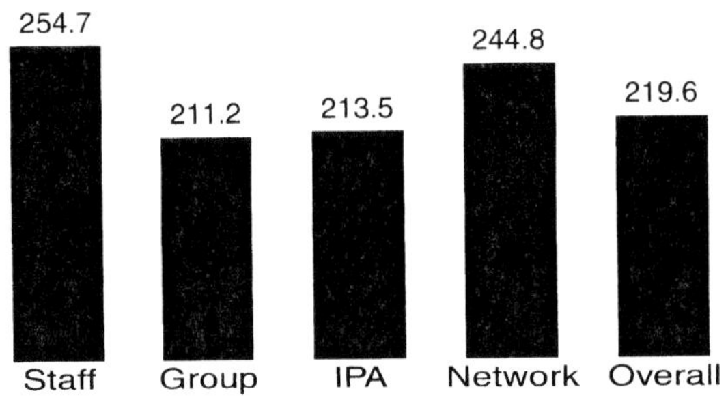

Source: Novartis (1997). The Novartis Pharmacy Benefit Report: Facts & Figures, 1997 Edition. East Hanover, NJ: Novartis Pharmaceuticals Corporation, p. 30. Reprinted by permission.

Non-compliance appears to be an issue here. Numerous studies have found that a significant number of patients do not fill their prescriptions, while other patients who do obtain the prescribed drugs fail to complete the course of therapy as directed or otherwise use their drugs inappropriately (Leibowitz, Manning & Newhouse, 1985; OIG, 1997; PhRMA, 1997). . . .

Regulatory Mandates

The primary legal rationale for government regulation of MCOs is to protect consumers. Some states also have acted to protect the economic and professional interests of certain providers, as through the adoption of "any willing provider" legislation. A few states also have used narrower "any willing provider" laws to preserve access to services in clinically underserved areas (Ladenheim & Markus, 1995).

Regulation is an important supplement to the limited contractual remedies available to enrollees in managed care plans. Consumers can appeal through established grievance procedures when they have disputes over coverage, quality or access; however, this avenue of redress is costly and time-consuming, and often is not well-understood by enrollees (Families USA Foundation, 1996).

Support for Regulation: A number of managed care organizations agree with consumer advocates on the need for national standards for managed care to eliminate what has been called a "crazy quilt" of regulations at the state and federal level. In September 1997, for example, managed care providers Kaiser Permanente, New York's HIP Health Insurance Plans, and the Group Health Cooperative of Puget Sound joined with the consumer advocacy groups Families USA and the American Association of Retired Persons in calling for 18 principles of consumer protection to be embodied in national standards. The principles cover assured choice of health plan and of primary care physician, as well as "prudent layperson" language that would require coverage of emergency care when a patient reasonably believes it is needed. The principles specifically call for an objective process to review new drugs, devices and therapies (Aston, 1997).

This initiative differs from the self-regulation approach favored by other managed care organizations and the American Association of Health Plans, which argues that "rather than micromanage, government should provide a framework in which the marketplace can play its proven role in driving innovation and continual improvement in quality of care" (Aston, 1997).

The advantage of federally enforced standards over industry self-policing, according to a spokesman for Families USA, is that "every American, no matter where they live, no matter what plan they're in, no matter who pays for their health services, [would] have the protection of legally enforceable standards for which they can seek real remedies" (Aston, 1997). Rodwin (1996) argues that a consumer voice is needed to advance both governmental and non-governmental oversight.

Limitations on Regulation: The federal Employee Retirement Income Security Act (ERISA) limits the ability of states to regulate employment-based managed care plans by preempting state laws that relate to employee health plans. Consequently, state standards for plan solvency, quality and grievance processes cannot be applied directly to ERISA-covered plans (i.e., those that are self-funded). Critics have charged that this creates incentives for employers to self-fund to avoid state regulation. Because the courts have not yet made it clear exactly what activities constitute the business of insurance that states may regulate, there may be ERISA challenges to some of the states' current regulatory activities.

Measuring Quality and Outcomes

Miller and Luft (1997) reviewed 15 studies of quality of care in managed care arrangements and found equal numbers of statistically significant positive and negative results for HMO performance. Because of these mixed results, they concluded that "HMO proponents and opponents alike can find support for their position on the quality of care. . . . The results show something that is simple, obvious, and yet sometimes underemphasized: HMOs produce better, the same, and worse quality of care, depending on the particular organization and particular disease." . . .

Lohr (1997) identifies three problem areas that need to be addressed by quality measures: "technical and interpersonal competence; overuse of unnecessary and inappropriate services; and underuse (or lack of access to) needed and appropriate services." She adds that the financial incentives in fee-for-service care tend to make overuse the principal problem, while managed care contains incentives that could lead to underuse (with competence an issue of equal concern in all systems), and argues that external quality standards and measurement programs are essential in monitoring plan performance in these areas. . . .

A number of organizations are attempting to develop some sort of universally accepted quality assurance measures. Pharmaceutical outcomes research holds the potential to demonstrate that a well-managed prescription drug benefit that ensures appropriate use of pharmacotherapies improves patient outcomes and contributes to overall cost savings (Mullins, Baldwin & Perfetto, 1996; Armstead, Elstein & Gorman, 1995; Benjamin, Perfetto & Greene, 1995). Models used in such research include decision analysis, cost-effectiveness analysis, cost-consequences modeling, and assessment of humanistic outcomes such as functional status, quality of life, and patient satisfaction (Stergachis, 1995).

Information/Data Systems

In the past, large state and federal databases tracked patients' use of services, outcomes, and health care costs. Today, managed care organizations maintain information on patients but may not report it consistently (Palumbo & Mullins, 1997). Each of the major managed care organizations has its own unique database. Some databases contain millions of claims records that must be manipulated to produce usable analytic files. Moreover, there are no industry-wide standardized data collection systems that allow managed care plans to compare many types of data to each other or to data from other providers, although numerous committees and task forces have been convened to address this issue. Data comparisons across managed care plans or between those plans and other providers thus may be misleading.

IPAs and network model HMOs have many of the same data limitations as do indemnity plans, but they have the ability to sample their members and to supplement their claims data with medical record and survey data. Group and staff model HMOs often have detailed medical record data because of their ability to centralize and share medical records among all panel providers, but they often have limited payment or encounter data (Swindle, Beattie & Barnett, 1996).

In the public sector, the Omnibus Budget Reconciliation Act of 1993 directed DHHS to establish and operate a clearinghouse to collect information on services delivered to Medicare and Medicaid beneficiaries. The clearinghouse also is to maintain health insurance information on individuals covered under employer group health plans. To facilitate the collection of data, legislation creating comprehensive data systems mandates the submission of detailed information by hospitals, insurers and other providers. Data collected usually includes type of services provided, charges, patient information and outcomes, and type of insurance coverage.

In the private sector, pharmaceutical manufacturers that have forged alliances with PBMs have gained access to data concerning who is using certain drugs, how often, and at what volume. This type of utilization information can be extremely useful to pharmaceutical companies when forming their marketing efforts (OIG, 1997).

In its report of a recent investigation, the DHHS Office of Inspector General said that data on service utilization do not flow as readily in managed care plans as in fee-for-service systems. This is at least partially due to the fact that in fee-for-service care, data are captured in individual claims, which are submitted for payment at the time services are provided. In managed care, however, purchasers pay a capitated rate for services not yet provided. Without specific data collection requirements, providers may lack the incentive to accurately report individual-level data on services delivered, since payment is not linked to documentation of such care (OIG, 1997).

Analysts agree that, over time, competitive pressures from some purchasers are likely to force managed care plans to produce some kinds of comparable information, such as HEDIS data and financial statements. Over time, too, researchers will improve methods for generating data that are accurate, meaningful, and comparable across model types and individual organizations (OIG, 1997). . . .

DISCUSSION AND RECOMMENDATIONS

The results of the study highlight both the challenge and the urgency of additional research on the impact of managed care on the pharmaceutical marketplace. . . .

Miller and Luft (1997), reporting mixed results in a survey of 37 managed care performance studies, caution that while recent research provides "useful results for health policymakers, analysts, and consumers, . . . interpreting and generalizing from the available studies is very difficult." Few analysts have attempted or been able to address the larger questions raised by the advent of managed care. In fact the published research findings to date clearly are only a starting point for the work that needs to be done in light of the increasingly competitive marketplace and changes in the delivery of health care.

Gray and Donald (1997) point to two areas of difficulty in this regard: (1) the difficulty most decisionmakers have in finding good quality evidence when and where they need it, and (2) the variable quality of research findings, and the difficulty most decisionmakers have in discriminating among them. Miller and Luft (1997) concluded that "for decisionmakers, some evidence is better than no evidence, but the policy debate is taking place with evidence that is quite limited, given the importance of the debate."

These potential problems notwithstanding, arriving at answers to the research and evaluation questions posed in the framework is a critical step with significant implications for a variety of stakeholder groups:

Government: Federal, state and local governments have multiple roles in relation to the issues raised by the study. As research funder, for example, government can create an open, ordered process for defining the questions that should be addressed in future research solicitations. As regulator, government has a need for the kinds of information that will help assess the effects of changing marketplace organizations and how those effects can be either promoted or mitigated through government interventions. As purchaser of services, government shares the interest of other purchasers in receiving optimal results, in terms of cost-efficiency and quality, for the health benefit dollars expended.

Pharmaceutical Manufacturers: Drugmakers have an obvious interest in, and are active sponsors of, pharmacoeconomic studies of particular drug products, as well as of studies that assess the climate for product introduction and regulation. Manufacturers also have a pressing interest in the effects of pharmacy benefit managers, health maintenance organizations, preferred provider organizations and other delivery arrangements; their effect on choice of drugs to treat specific conditions; the development and effects of disease management programs; the effects and effectiveness of provider and patient education campaigns, and the like.

Purchasers: Organizations covered by the Employee Retirement Income Security Act (ERISA), traditional insurers, employers, consumers, and other parties that purchase health care benefits–including pharmacotherapies and related services–share with government-as-payer an interest in purchasing good quality care at a reasonable cost. This translates into an urgent need for research results that elucidate the immediate and long-term effects of various changes in service organization and delivery systems, as exemplified by managed care.

Providers: Medical and pharmacy organizations and other provider groups have a stake in research that helps explain the forces changing traditional professional practice patterns. In essence, they need to understand the impact of managed care on how health professionals do what they do. This kind of information makes it possible not only to shape current practice patterns in positive ways, but also to project developing trends that will shape the future of the health professions.

Health Centers: The implications of managed care for reimbursement patterns, graduate and continuing health professions education, development and adoption of clinical practice guidelines, and the like, all make research into managed care a central issue for academic health centers.

Managed Care Organizations: As organizations at the center of the health care delivery revolution described in the literature reviewed for this study, MCOs have a compelling interest in fostering research to assist in selecting management techniques and approaches that advance their stated goals of concurrent cost containment and quality improvement. As Bernstein and Bernstein (1997) put it, "by building bridges with (and within) the research community, managed care organizations and researchers can pool their data and expertise to address these questions and help shape the future health care delivery system."

REFERENCES

Armstead RC, Elstein P & Gorman J (1995). HCFA's Plans for Assuring Managed Care Quality: Toward a 21st Century Quality-Measurement System for Managed Care Organizations. *Health Care Financing Review* Summer.

Armstrong EP (1996). Disease State Management and Its Influence on Health Systems Today. *Drug Benefit Trends* 8(7): 18-20, 25, 29.

Aston G (1997). Discord on Managed Care Standards. *American Medical News* 40(38): 1, 34-35.

Benjamin KL, Perfetto EM & Greene RJ (1995). Public Policy and the Application of Outcomes Assessment: Paradigms versus Politics. *Medical Care* 33(4): AS299-AS306.

Berndt ER (1994). *Uniform Pharmaceutical Pricing: An Economic Analysis.* Washington, DC: American Enterprise Institute Press.

Bernstein AB & Bernstein J (1996). HMOs and Health Services Research: The Penalty of Taking the Lead. *Medical Care Research and Review* 53:S18-S43.

Bloom BS & Fendrick AM (1996). The Tension Between Cost Containment and the Underutilization of Effective Health Services. *International Journal of Technology Assessment in Health Care* 12(1): 1-8.

Boston Consulting Group (BCG) (1996). *Sustaining Innovation in U.S. Pharmaceuticals: Intellectual Property Protection and the Role of Patents.* Boston, MA: BCG.

Boston Consulting Group (BCG) (1993). *The Contribution of Pharmaceutical Companies: What's at Stake for America.* Boston, MA: BCG.

Buchanan JL, Leibowitz A & Keesey J (1996). Medicaid Health Maintenance Organizations–Can They Reduce Program Spending? *Medical Care* 34(3):249-263.

Christensen DB & Fassett WE (1996). Understanding Capitation and Pharmaceutical Care. *Journal of the American Pharmaceutical Association* NS36(6):374-380.

Colorado Task Force on Consumer Access to Prescription Drugs (Colorado) (1994). *A Report on Consumer Access to Prescription Drugs.* Denver, CO: Colorado HCP&L.

Comanor WS & Schweitzer SO (1995). Pharmaceuticals. In W Adams & JW Brock (eds.) *The Structure of American Industry.* Englewood Cliffs, NJ: Prentice-Hall, 177-196.

Curtiss FR (1986). Methods of Providing Prescription Drug Benefits in Health Plans. *American Journal of Hospital Pharmacy* 43: 2428-2434.

Cutler DM & Sheiner L (1997). *Managed Care and the Growth of Medical Expenditures.* Washington, DC: National Bureau of Economic Research.

DeNoon DJ (1996). Drug Companies' Control of Pharmacy Benefits: Conflict of Interest. *AIDS Weekly Plus* June 3;4.

DiMasi JA, Grabowski H & Vernon J (1995). R&D Costs, Innovative Output and Firm Size in the Pharmaceutical Industry. *International Journal of the Economics of Business* 2(2):201-219.

Epstein RS & McGlynn MG (1997). Disease Management: What Is It? *Disease Management & Health Outcomes* 1(1): 3-10.

Etheredge L (1995). *Pharmacy Benefit Management: The Right Rx?* Washington, DC: Health Insurance Reform Project, The George Washington University.

Families USA Foundation (1996). *HMO Consumers at Risk: States to the Rescue.* Washington, DC: The Foundation.

Fillenbaum GG, Hanlon JT, Corder EH et al. (1993). Prescription and Nonprescription Drug Use Among Black and White Community-Residing Elderly. *American Journal of Public Health* 83(11):1577-1582.

Gagnon JP (1996). Future Partnerships within the Drug Distribution System. *A Pharmacist's Guide to Principles and Practices of Managed Care Pharmacy* 145-155.

Genuardi JS, Stiller JM & Trapnell GR (1996). Changing Prescription Drug Sector: New Expenditure Methodologies. *Health Care Financing Review* 17(3):191-205.

Grabowski HG (1994). *Health Reform and Pharmaceutical Innovation.* Washington, DC: American Enterprise Institute.

Grabowski HG (1988). Medicaid Patients' Access to New Drugs. *Health Affairs* 7:102-114.

Grabowski H & Vernon (1990). A New Look at the Returns and Risks to Pharmaceutical R&D. *Management Science* 36:804-821.

Grabowski H & Vernon (1994). Returns to R&D on New Drug Introductions in the 1980s. *Journal of Health Economics* 13:383-406.

Gray JAM & Donald A (1997). Policy and Quality Standards. *Evidence-Based Health Policy and Management.* 1(1):iii-iv.

Gross DJ (1995). *Issues Related to the Federal Government Drug Payment Policies in the Reformed Health Care Environment: Final Report to HCFA.* Washington, DC: KPMG Peat Marwick-Policy Economics Group, September 5.

Hahn BA (1995). Children's Health: Racial and Ethnic Differences in the Use of Prescription Medicines. *Pediatrics* 95(5):727-732.

Health Care Financing Administration (HCFA) (1997). Homepage. World Wide Web: http://www.hcfa.gov.

Hellinger FJ (1995). Selection Bias in HMOs and PPOs; A Review of the Evidence. *Inquiry* 32:135-142.

Horn SD, Sharkey PD, Tracy DM et al. (1996). Intended and Unintended Consequences of HMO Cost-Containment Strategies: Results from the Managed Care Outcomes Project. *The American Journal of Managed Care* II(3):253-264.

Hux JE & Naylor CD (1994). Drug Prices and Third Party Payment: Do They Influence Medication Selection? *Pharmacoeconomics* 5(4):343-350.

Iglehart J (1994b). Health Policy Report: The Struggle Between Managed Care and Fee-For-Service Practice. *The New England Journal of Medicine* 331(1):63-67.

Institute of Medicine (1997a). *Managing Managed Care: Quality Improvement in Behavioral Health*. Washington, DC: National Academy Press.

Institute of Medicine (1997b). *Medicare: A Strategy for Quality Assurance* (K Lohr, ed.). Washington, DC: National Academy Press.

Jensen GA, Morrisey MA, Gaffney S, et al. (1997). The New Dominance of Managed Care: Insurance Trends in the 1990s. *Health Affairs* 16(1):125-136.

Johnson NE (1995). A Primer on Pharmacoeconomics. *The Journal of Outcomes Management* Fall:8-9.

Johnson RE, Goodman MJ, Hornbrook MC & Eldredge MB (1997). The Impact of Increasing Patient Prescription Drug Cost Sharing on Therapeutic Classes of Drugs Received and on the Health Status of Elderly HMO Members. *Health Services Research* 32(1):103-122.

Kitchner M (1992). Managed Care Lexicon. *Business & Health (Special Report: Managed Care Comes to Prescription Drugs)* April:12-13.

Knickman JR, Hughes RG, Taylor H et al. (1996). Tracking Consumers' Reactions to the Changing Health Care System: Early Indicators. *Health Affairs* 15(2): 21-32.

Knowlton CH & Knapp DA (1994). Community Pharmacists Help HMO Cut Drug Costs. *American Pharmacy* NS34(1):36-42.

KPMG Peat Marwick (1996). *Integrated Patient Care: Managing Health Care Costs, Maximizing Health Care Value and Quality*. Washington, DC: KPMG Peat Marwick, April.

Ladenheim K & Markus A (1995). *State Any Willing Provider Laws and Related Activities: Implications for Technology*. Washington, DC: Intergovernmental Health Policy Project, The George Washington University.

Lasagna L, ed. (1994). *Health Care Reforms and the Role of the Pharmaceutical Industry (Proceedings of a European Workshop)*. European Commission, September 16-17.

Leibowitz A, Manning WG & Newhouse JP (1985). The Demand for Prescription Drugs as a Function of Cost-Sharing. *Social Science and Medicine* 21(10): 1063-1069.

McGinley L (1997). Seniors' Dropout Rates Vary Widely at HMOs. *The Wall Street Journal* Dec. 5:B10.

Miller RH & Luft HS (1997). Does Managed Care Lead to Better or Worse Quality of Care? *Health Affairs* 16(5):7-24.

Miller RH & Luft HS (1994). Managed Care Plan Performance Since 1980: A Literature Analysis. *Journal of the American Medical Association* 271(19): 1512-1519.

Moore J (1996). *The Pharmaceutical Industry*. Washington, DC: National Health Policy Forum, The George Washington University.

Mullins CD, Baldwin R & Perfetto EM (1996). What are Outcomes? *Journal of the American Pharmaceutical Association* January.

Nagy K (1995). Pharmaceutical Industry Buys Into Managed Care. *Journal of the National Cancer Institute* 87:1278-1279.

Nash (1995). Why Today's Health Care Requires Integration. *The Journal of Outcomes Management* (Special Issue) 2:4-6.

Novartis (1997a). *Pharmacy Benefit Report: Facts and Figures.* East Hanover, NJ: Novartis, Inc.

Novartis (1997b). *Pharmacy Benefit Report: Trends and Forecasts.* East Hanover, NJ: Novartis, Inc.

Office of the Inspector General (OIG) (1997). *Experiences of Health Maintenance Organizations with Pharmacy Benefit Management Companies (OEI-01-95-00110).* Washington, DC: OIG, April.

Pharmaceutical Research and Manufacturers of America (PhRMA) (1997). 1997 Industry Profile. Washington, DC: PhRMA.

Pollard MR (1990). Managed Care and a Changing Pharmaceutical Industry. *Health Affairs* 9(3):55-65.

Reeder CE & Nelson AA (1985). The Differential Impact of Copayment on Drug Use in a Medicaid Population. *Inquiry* 22(Winter):396-403.

Rodwin MA (1996). Consumer Protection and Managed Care: The Need for Organized Consumers. *Health Affairs* 15(3): 110-123.

Rosenbaum S & Richards TB (1996). Medicaid Managed Care and Public Health Policy. *Journal of Public Health Management and Practice* Summer.

Rucker TD (1983). Drug-Utilization Review: Moving Toward an Effective and Safe Model. In JP Morgan & DV Kagan (eds.) *Society and Medication: Conflicting Signals for Prescribers and Patients.* Lexington, MA: Lexington Books.

Schulman KA, Rubenstein LE, Abernethy DR et al. (1996). The Effect of Pharmaceutical Benefits Managers: Is It Being Evaluated? *Annals of Internal Medicine* 124(10):906-913.

Schweitzer SO, Salehi H & Boling N (1985). The Social Drug Lag: An Examination of Pharmaceutical Approval Delays in Medicaid Formularies. *Social Science and Medicine* 21(10):1077-1082.

Schweitzer SO & Shiota SR (1992). Access and Cost Implications of State Limitations on Medicaid Reimbursement for Pharmaceuticals. *Annual Review of Public Health* 13:399-410.

Short PF (1996). *Medicaid's Role in Insuring Low-Income Women.* New York, NY: The RAND Corp.

Shulman S, Healy E & Lasagna L, eds. (1997). PBMs: Reshaping the Pharmaceutical Distribution Network. *Journal of Pharmaceutical Marketing and Management* (Fall issue).

Shulman SR & Brown JS (1995). The Food and Drug Administration's Early Access and Fast-Track Approval Initiatives: How Have They Worked? *Food and Drug Law Journal* 50:503-531.

Soumerai SB, Avorn J & Ross-Degnan D (1987). Payment Restrictions for Prescription Drugs Under Medicaid. *The New England Journal of Medicine* 317(9):550-556.

Soumerai SB & Lipton HL (1995). Computer-Based Drug-Utilization Review–Risk, Benefit, or Boondoggle? *The New England Journal of Medicine* 332(24): 1641-1645.

Soumerai SB, Ross-Degnan D, Fortess EE & Abelson J (1993). A Critical Analysis of Studies of State Drug Reimbursement Policies: Research in Need of Discipline. *The Milbank Quarterly* 71(2):217-252.

Stergachis A (1995). Overview of Cost-Consequence Modeling in Outcomes Research. *Pharmacotherapy* 15(5):405-425.

Summers KH & Gumbhir AK (1991). The Expected Impact of Managed Health Care Organizations on the Research-Intensive U.S. Pharmaceutical Industry. *Journal of Pharmaceutical Marketing & Management* 5(3):65-77.

Swindle RW, Beattie MC & Barnett PG (1996). The Quality of Cost Data. *Medical Care Supplement* 34(3):MS83-MS90.

Taylor AK, Beauregard KM & Vistnes JP (1995). Who Belongs to HMOs: A Comparison of Fee-for-Service versus HMO Enrollees. *Medical Care Research & Review* 52(3):389-407.

Vogenberg (1997a). Managed Health Care: A Review. *Hospital Pharmacy* 32(7): 975-982.

Vogenberg (1997b). Medicare and Managed Health Care. *Hospital Pharmacy* 32(10): 1324-1331.

Ware JE, Bayliss MS, Rogers WH et al. (1996). Differences in Four-Year Health Outcomes for Elderly and Poor, Chronically Ill Patients Treated in HMO and Fee-For-Service Systems. *Journal of the American Medical Association* 276(13): 1039-1047.

Weiner JP, Lyles A, Steinwachs D & Hall KC (1991). Impact of Managed Care on Prescription Drug Use. *Health Affairs* 10(1):140-154.

Zimmerman D, Collins T, Lipowski E et al. (1994). *Guidelines for Estimating the Impact of Medicaid DUR*. Silver Spring, MD: Shepard Patterson, Inc., for the Health Care Financing Administration, USDHHS.

MEMBERS OF THE ADVISORY PANEL

Opinions and recommendations offered by members of the Advisory Panel are their own and do not necessarily represent those of the organizations with which the are (or were) affiliated.

James R. Allen, M.D., M.P.H.
Vice President
Science, Technology and Public
Health
American Medical Association

Lynn A. Bosco, M.D., M.P.H.
Pharmaceutical Outcomes
Research Program
Agency for Health Care Policy
& Research

Calvin J. Anthony, Pharm.D.
Executive Vice President
National Community Pharmacy
Association

Laurie Beth Burke, R.Ph., M.P.H.
Senior Regulations Research
Officer
Food and Drug Administration

Patricia J. Byrns, M.D.
Director, Division of Drugs &
Technology Standards
American Medical Association

Cheryl Austein Casnoff
Director, Division of Public
Health Policy
U.S. Department of Health &
Human Services

David Clark, R.Ph., M.B.A.
Senior Advisor, Office
of Managed Care
Health Care Financing
Administration

Burke Fishburn, M.P.P.
Senior Policy Analyst
Food & Drug Policy
U.S. Department of Health &
Human Services

Thomas R. Fulda
Program Director, DUR
United States Pharmacopeia

Jean-Paul Gagnon, R.Ph., Ph.D.
Director, Health Economics Policy
Hoechst Marion Roussel, Inc.

Linda F. Golodner
President
National Consumers League

Kathleen Gondek, Ph.D.
Office of Science
Health Care Financing
Administration

Henry Grabowski, Ph.D.
Professor and Chairman
Department of Economics
Duke University

Charles R. Grezlak, Ph.D.
Executive Director
Government Affairs and Policy
U.S. Human Health Division
Merck & Co., Inc.

David J. Gross, Ph.D.
Senior Policy Advisor
American Association
of Retired Persons

Eric Katz, J.D.
Director of Research Partnerships
Health Care Financing
Administration

Arthur Lawrence, M.D., M.P.H.
Assistant Surgeon General
Office of the Assistant Secretary
for Health
U.S. Department of Health &
Human Services

Helene L. Lipton, Ph.D.
Professor of Pharmacy
& Medicine
Institute for Health Policy Studies
UCLA School of Medicine

Lucinda L. Maine, Ph.D.
Senior Vice President
for Professional Affairs
American Pharmaceutical
Association

Julie Matsumoto, M.S.T.H.
Consumer Advocate for
Los Angeles County, CA

Patrick L. McKercher, R.Ph.,
Ph.D.
Executive Director/Research
Professor
Center on Drugs and Public
Policy
College of Pharmacy
University of Maryland at
Baltimore

Michael Miller, M.D.
Director, Federal Relations
Pfizer, Inc.

Louis Morris, Ph.D.
Branch Chief, Division of Drug
Marketing,
Advertising & Communication
U.S. Food and Drug
Administration

(former) Mark Novitch, M.D.,
(Principal Investigator)
Professor of Health Care Sciences
The George Washington
University
Medical Center

Francis B. Palumbo, Ph.D., J.D.
Associate Director
Center on Drugs and Public
Policy
College of Pharmacy
University of Maryland
at Baltimore

Peter M. Penna, Pharm.D.
Vice President, Managed
Pharmacy
CIGNA Healthcare

Gary S. Persinger
Vice President
Research and Information
Services
Pharmaceutical Research
and Manufacturers of America

Michael Pollard, J.D., M.P.H.
Michaels, Wishner & Bonner

T.Donald Rucker, Ph.D.
Professor Emeritus
of Pharmacy Administration
University of Illinois at Chicago

Claudia Schur, Ph.D.
Deputy Director, Center
for Health Affairs
Project HOPE

Stuart O. Schweitzer, Ph.D.
Professor of Health Economics
Department of Health Services
UCLA School of Public Health

David G. Schulke
Director, Policy and Regulatory
Affairs
American Pharmaceutical
Association

Kevin A. Schulman, M.D.
Director, Clinical Economics
Research Unit
Assistant Professor of Medicine
Georgetown University Medical
School

Robert C. Seidman, M.P.H.
Director of Pharmacy
Blue Cross of California

Sheila R. Shulman, L.L.B.,
M.P.H.
Assistant Director
Tufts Center for the Study of
Drug Development

Betsy L. Sleath, Ph.D., R.Ph.
Assistant Professor, School of
Pharmacy
University of North Carolina at
Chapel Hill

Janice Whitehouse
Manager, National Managed
Pharmacy Program
General Motors Corporation

(former) Bonnie B. Wilford
Senior Research Scientist and
Director, Pharmaceutical Policy
Project
The George Washington
University
Medical Center

Karen Williams
President
National Pharmaceutical Council

Raymond L. Woosley, M.D.,
Ph.D.
Professor and Chairman
Department of Pharmacology
Georgetown University Medical
Center

Index

Page numbers followed by f indicate figures; page numbers followed by t indicate tables.